Coping

Coping

A Black Cancer Patients Observation

Warren G. H. Fisher, Jr., USN (RET)

Writers Club Press
San Jose New York Lincoln Shanghai

Coping
A black cancer patients observation

Writers Club Press
an imprint of iUniverse.com, Inc.

For information address:
iUniverse.com, Inc.
620 North 48th Street, Suite 201
Lincoln, NE 68504-3467
www.iuniverse.com

Photograph contributors:
Warren G.H. Fisher Sr., aka Fabulous Fisher
Warren G. H. Fisher Jr., dba Warren Electric
Irene W. Fisher
Frances E. Fisher

ISBN: 0-595-13543-9

Printed in the United States of America

Contents

Introduction xi

As a Black, life is complicated 1

Hot Days, Cool Nights..4

Note to Reader 10

The Adventure Begins 12

Coping 14

Who Prepared Me for the Transplant?....................................20

Good Morning America 21

Recovery! 23

I Wonder 27

Snoopy, Welcome Home 31

A Lighter Side: Food to Eat, Things to Do, Places to See 35

To the Beach...37

What do I Think About All This?..39

It's Getting Tough, But You Must Be Tougher.........................41

The Norm 43

Responsibility 44

This Is a Growing Experience 46

Believing In Yourself...47

Heroes 49

Destined to Fail 51

Fighting Negative Thinking 55

Moving Through the Turbulence 59

Still Writing 62

Family 63

Happy Birthday 65

Changes Through a Passing of Time 66

Demons 70

Adolescence 75

Ethnic Cleansing 77

A Slave 79

A Black Mans Dilemma 81

Niggar 82

Black Man's Tears 84

The Interview 86

The Tickets..90

The Mystery Aircraft 98

Vacationing in Greece 105

Black Cowboys 107

Always Striving to Improve 110

Discrimination Still Linger 113

News Flash 117

About the Military 119

Black Sailors 122

Advancing Upward 126

Black Sailors Today 130

Memories 131

Home 139

Traveling Through Time..142

Welcome to Warren Electric 144

Business 147

Competition 150

Satisfied Customers 152

Self...154

Faith...156

My First Christmas 159
Whew! Time Really Flies 160
Challenge 162
A Hero is Gone..166
It's Tough Trying to Survive in Today's World 170
Welcome to the Café 175
Through the Eyes of Dreamers 178
Am I My Mother's Child 180

LIST OF ILLUSTRATIONS

meandtom 31

jims grandkids 32

gene and lina 63

african_family...64

leanna wedding dress 64

warrenas baby...66

shaw church 66

museum printer 86

black_cowgirl 108

black footballteam 110

curtis jiggsreedsr 111

emschool 123

granddaddy and grandmother warren 132

grandpoppas farm..135

daddy donaldjoann...139

daddymomma students...140

warren in native dress 141

meandsandra 152

warrens birthday 160

family 161

tribal dancers 167

black_cafe..175

the dreamer 178

blacklady 179
warren greek restauranr..180
camera 183

INTRODUCTION

This is based on my experience of having gone through the Veteran Administration Hospital Bone Marrow Transplant program. I also speak of my experience in life and my religious beliefs which strengthen me as I went through the program. I talk about military life. I joined the Navy in August 1962 as a recruit and retired October 1983 as a Chief Petty Officer. I was stationed on numerous ships including the USS MIDWAY CVA 41(homeport Alameda California), USS CREE ATF 84(Home ported San Diego, California), USS PAGE FFG 5(Home ported Athens, Greece). I also serviced at a host of shore duty stations Boston Naval Yard (Boston Mass.), Norfolk Naval Shipyard (Norfolk Va.) Fleet Support Office(Athens Greece). I attended 10 or more Navy training schools.

I was diagnosed with cancer by the Navy, which started my chemotherapy treatment in 1993; then all the military medical facilities closed. There wasn't a military medical facility (available for retirees and their families) within 60 miles. My doctors and I were upset because as a retired navy veteran we felt I should have received better treatment. Many forget that medical was one of the benefits promised all service people for sacrifices made and now it appears we are ignored for political reason. There are civilian hospitals nearby, however they wouldn't treat me unless I had insurance. When the military hospitals closed and I had no place to go, (my Doctor at Oaknoll Hospital advised me and gave me a letter of introduction) I took my medical record to the VA Clinic in Martinez, California; they immediately started me on chemotherapy and eventually scheduled me for the Bone Marrow Transplant program. The VA program insured that I got excellent service and all my benefits. Support I should have gotten from the Navy (Military). Because I'm Black I also write about the Black experience. As a Black cancer patient I must deal with the negative images created of Blacks as well as the discomforts of cancer. I believe that many attempt to ignore us and that includes many Blacks, instead of struggle for change. I believe the future is now and nothing positive will happen unless we make change. ARE YOU READY?

Chief Warren G. H. Fisher Jr. USN (RET)

As a Black, Life is Complicated

Many ask when you write why talk about everything? I was raised in a Black community where I was taught values. Now I'm grown and out in the world and things aren't what I was taught now I find that as a Black man there is a separate set of rules. Myself I talk about everything because here in America many things from different directions confront our lives as Blacks.

I've seen countries totally destroyed and over a short period of time they have made a miraculous recovery, but a hundred years after slavery Blacks still have not been allowed to make any major impact on the American economy. As a cancer patient people say I should talk just about cancer, and I ask why? As a Black I've seen the ugly and complicated side of America. I say we don't have to live like this and I want to see a change.

Sometimes I wonder if we should have some type civil war or a political revolution. What we do need is a Black Industrial revolution. With a industrial revolution a market is create for our products and services, like the computer we need to create a product or service that everyone feels they need. Something that we can push for years. It doesn't have to be one thing; it can also be a group of things. We train and educate and we are still not pulled into this new political or economic climate. So we have to be creative. I see articles about Black workers and how we are now getting jobs but there is nothing about a Black Business market. What is this all about? Are you now saying that after 100 years we now qualify for technical jobs and that is all? With a true industrial revolution an atmosphere is created where everyone feels nothing will happen without your products and services, and that's from labor to management.

Everyone talk about how we're not doing anything, but I see hate crimes on the increase. Example—in Chicago a Black educator was shot and killed while walking his kids. Another educated Black has been lost to hate and his death is a warning message for his kids. You constantly read of more white hate groups being developed and the same people attempting to hold Blacks back are funding them. Many ask is there any hope? I say yes, but you must make the change because it is obvious no one else will.

How can there be change when the Black male is put against the Black female. Here is a very unstable situation. The atmosphere where men wear clothing that falls off them. The atmosphere is created where drug use is normal. Or the picture where men are walking with their head hanging down and they are dragging their feet.

There is a picture of low esteem, and loss of confidence being created in the Black community. We are not creating this picture, it's the picture created by others. I look back at my return from the Bone Marrow Transplant and seeing the surprise on everyone's face. Many thought I was going to die during the process. Hey, no such luck. As a cancer patient going through the transplant it is really tough. As a Black cancer patient it is even tougher because there is a lack of confidence on the part of many. It's amazing how that lack of confidence can reach from the community to the medical ward.

Trained in the Black community, having worked for Black businesses, all these false label placed on Blacks are misplaced. These companies helped me get to where I am today. One such company was Superior Engineering in San Diego, California. They also had an office and manu-facturing facility in Norfolk Virginia. This was a large company that built and installed computer systems for the government. Black businesses are out there large and small, but everyone will say that they can't find us. For us this is bad. This means we must work 3 times as hard to find customers and investors.

So for a Black, life is complicated. Just talking about one thing when talking about cancer is impossible, because to get through everything I must look at where I came from, where I've been, what I've gone through, and where I want to go. I want to create my future and not have my future created by others.

HOT DAYS, COOL NIGHTS

Those hot days on the Aircraft Carrier in the engine room. This was the days before good insulation. Here there was no air conditioning, here your only air supply was from massive blowers or what many would call piped in air. Here the temperature was very hot, 120 degrees plus and because of that extreme heat a special room or booth was built in the space so that when you weren't working or checking machinery there was somewhere comfortable for you to go, and you drank iced tea by the bucket. In those early days of Ship Board life on combat ships there was very little insulation on hot pipe and no luxury like Air Conditioning in engineering or the crews living quarters. Cruising in the south pacific the weather outside was hot and below decks it was worse. Relief comes when you leave your work space and go to the mess decks, here the air was cooled by force draft blowers, or you could venture out to the ships main deck catching the breeze as the ship glides across the water. At noon looking for a cool place to take a nap I would venture up to the flight deck where airmen are loading bombs on planes getting ready for air strikes, and there I would lay on those bombs the breeze caressing my face as I slept. At night to keep cool I slept under blower vents.

One pleasure on those hot days was the salad bar meals on the mess decks. Here you could get watermelon, mangos, apricots and plenty of Kool-Aid to help you keep cool. Everyone attempts to find ways to make themselves comfortable. Being a sailor who has served in both the Pacific and North Atlantic fleets on those hot days in the Pacific I would think of those cool days on the North Atlantic, and the Chesapeake bay, the smell of fresh lobsters, crabs, and shrimp. Oh those cool days.

The ship was now in the middle of its 6-month cruise and we were off the coast of Vietnam. During the day I worked in distribution where part of my responsibility was being able to work on any electrical equipment in engineering. My workstation is #1 electrical switchboard group, which is 5 decks below the hanger bay. As an electrician my work area was #1 machinery group, which included #1 fire room, #1 engine room and associated machinery spaces. The work in these areas wasn't bad, but underway with all the boilers going, the temperature gets unbearable. With regular work, machinery watches and the heat, things can get pretty stressful. If something breaks down it has to be repaired immediately to maintain combat readiness, so it's not unusual for you to be working until 3 and 4 in the morning. I remember the phone ringing in the shop. It was the Chief Engineer, another pump burnt-out in the AFT fireroom, another hot space. The shop supervisor tells all the shop personnel that we must start repairs immediately. Where were those cool easy days?

For the engineers that worked in the Firerooms the temperature and working conditions were terrible. Not only did you have to deal with the heat from the boilers but also you were always checking the steam system for leaks because a pinhole size steam leak was enough to kill a man, and a ruptured steam pipe could kill everyone in the space. The fuel that was used to power these massive ships is genuine crude, which we called Black Oil, which came almost straight from the well. This stuff is like molasses. Working in the firerooms with the Black Oil and the soot from the boilers it wasn't unusual to see men cover from head to toe with dirt and oil their uniforms ruined. Because of all the dirt it wasn't unusual to see these men in the showers scrubbing each other.

Something you really hate is General Quarter's drills. Many times during a cruise, combat readiness inspections would be held, but this was a necessary event. For us engineer's general quarter was terrible especially in hot weather because much of your ventilation would be secured and if your battle station was a hot engineering space life became unbearable. The possibility of being in combat for us in engineering was scary because your only way out during an explosion or fire was through a steel 6" thick hatch 3 decks above, so you hope that in a real combat situation the repair party responsible for your space doesn't get wiped out. But, all that training paid off because once we had to actually go to general quarter because of an approaching unidentified aircraft. I think we set a record for securing the ship for combat. All stations were manned and ready in less than 3 minutes. While Ships Company was preparing for possible combat, you could feel that massive ship turning into the wind and hear the fighters being launched? I was 19 years old and scared to death. After the aircraft was intercepted our planes found it was an airliner and we were secured from General Quarters. During a cruise things would get hectic. Planes crashing into the flight deck, one airman was killed when another aircraft hit the plane he was taxiing to the side. A squadron commander was shot in the butt when his plane was hit by anti-aircraft. Life on the ship wasn't dull, but there was strict discipline.

After 3 years I was transferred to a Fleet Tug in San Diego. How did I get orders for a ship this size I'll never know? I went from the navy's largest ship, to one of the smallest. This ship had the capability of going anywhere in the world, with a crew of about 100 men crammed in two berthing compartments. Underway there never seem to be enough bunks. Many times you had to hot bunk with someone else. This meant that when a person got out of bed you sleep in his bed. During a long cruise it seemed like we were always running out of water for showers, when the fresh water supply was low everyone would take salt water showers and it wasn't bad. The summers were terrible because there was no air conditioning and during the winter we had poor heating. The crews' berthing was built over the fuel tanks. During the summer the fuel would expand and leak through the caps in the deck. You never forgot that fuel because when you entered berthing you would slide across the compartment to your bunk. We relied on an old donkey boiler for steam for heating, hot water, cooking, and laundry. The boiler also provided steam for the evaporator, which manufactured fresh water. The ships propulsion plant was 4 large motors powered by 4 large Diesel driven generators. For general lighting power was provided by 3 smaller diesel driven generators. Our main defense was a 3" gun on the bow.

Stationed here for three years was an experience. Many times you were frustrated because of the long working hours and the long periods away from family, but you were compensated with entertainment such as movies, in port we had family picnics and ships parties. Underway for the crew we were always having a BBQ on the ship's fantail. We never had lobster and crab like the larger ships, but we ate steaks as big as plates. The quality of your meals depended on your cook. The ship went through a lot of cooks. You had fun times; some of the guys went hunting in Alaska. I went shrimping in those Alaska chilly waters. I remember my first time getting seasick it was off the coast of northern California en route to Alaska. That was an experience I'll never forget because I awaken with my arm around the trash can. And you never forgot Petty Officer Browns beard being burnt off when he had a flair back in the ships boiler. We heard that explosion all through the ship. To us engineers it was funny because Brown had been told to always ventilate the boiler before lighting the fire. At times things were dangerous, a Boatswain Mates hand was caught in the towing machine crushing all his fingers, we were shot at by our own ships while towing targets, almost run over by larger ships in Vietnam, put out fires in Alaska. We towed disabled ships to Japan. We had liberty in Japan, Hong Kong, the Philippine Islands, and we were home ported during the fall season in Adak Alaska. Life wasn't boring because we did a lot of traveling for a ship that was smaller than a submarine. This may not be the Chesapeake Bay, but the pacific was a nice place to grow up.

Things weren't always hot; there were those rough seas in the Mediterranean. Here I was stationed on the USS Page FFG 5. Her and her five sister ships were some of smallest ships in the fleet. Propelled by 2 turbo supercharged boilers operating at 1200 pounds of steam pressure and a temperature of 900 degrees, with one propeller for propulsion these small Guided missile destroyers were true fleet gray hounds keeping up with any ship afloat. The Page had a top speed of 32 knots and on many occasions I saw her exceed that speed. During high speed operations to insure we maintain speed we engineers would transfer all unnecessary electrical power requirements to the ships diesels which meant the ships main engine got 100 percent steam. To many of us engineers hearing those turbo super chargers running was exciting, it sounded as if the ship was a living, breathing piece of machinery. To insure stability while operating in rough weather and the launching of missiles the ship was equipped with large computer controlled fins located below the ships water line. The fins were called ships fin stabilizers and when they weren't operating you would notice the difference in the ride of the ship. Even with all this you never forgot the rough weather because during high-speed runs no one was allowed out on the main deck all watertight doors and hatches were secured. We would hit those waves with such force the complete ship would shake. And on the bridge you would see water breaking over the bridge, the ship seemed more like a submarine. Below deck many of us senior engineers got very little sleep insuring all equipment ran smoothly. In the ships galley the cooks when not chasing pots and pans were constantly busy thinking of meals to feed those hungry appetites. These were exciting memories. I eventually moved my family to Virginia Beach, Virginia. The air there is cooled by a gentle breeze blowing off the Chesapeake Bay. During the day the beaches are filled with tourist getting tans and there's the sound of children playing in the surf. My wife Frances would go to the fish piers and buy fresh blue crabs, shrimp, and fish and make some fantastic gumbo. During my spare time I would be preparing for the 13-mile race at William and Mary College in Williamsburg. This was no time for McDonald's, Burger King or Pizza hut, during the day Frances prepares special meals with very little meat, but plenty of spaghetti, seafood, and fruit. I snacked on power bars and energy drinks developed by Frances. Starting at about 10 o'clock at night I would start my daily 10 mile run. I would be wearing almost nothing and sweating like mad. Frances would be riding her bicycle, coaching and setting the pace. During my daily run the police would drive by with words of encouragement. Sometime I laugh to myself because I remember running one evening and I came upon a lady running, surprising her she started screaming and I was so surprised that I started screaming with her. When we realized what had happened, we laughed and resumed our run.

To prepare for a race you practiced all the time, ate control diets, and exercised daily, because endurance is the important thing. But after those races my wife and I would have dinner at the nearest seafood restaurants and I would eat the night away. But after everything years later you still remembered those hot days in the Pacific and the cool night time breezes blowing off the Chesapeake.

NOTE TO READER

AS YOU READ YOU WILL FIND THAT I TALK ABOUT MY ILLNESS, MY EXPERIENCE AS A BLACK, THE PEOPLE THAT WORKED WITH ME, AND MY NEW FRIENDS INCLUDING THE ONE'S THAT DIED. YOU WILL FIND THAT MYSELF AND OTHER CANCER PATIENTS ARE FIGHTING TO SURVIVE AND IT'S A CONTINUING PROCESS. SOME OF US SUCCEED AND SOME FAIL.

SOME OF US FIND SUPPORT FROM FAMILY AND FRIENDS AND FOR MANY THERE IS NO SUPPORT EXCEPT FROM THEMSELVES. BUT WE FIGHT TO SURVIVE BECAUSE WE UNDERSTAND THE RESULT OF FAILURE.

MYSELF I BECOME UPSET WITH HEALTHY PEOPLE WHO SYSTEMATICALLY TRY TO KILL THEMSELVES THROUGH DRUG ABUSE, SOME ALLOW PEOPLE TO USE AND ABUSE THEM. THEY PUT THEMSELVES IN DANGEROUS POSITIONS LOOKING FOR EXCITEMENT KNOWING THAT THE END RESULTS COULD POSSIBLY KILL THEM. THEY HAVE SET NO GOALS AND WHEN YOU SPEAK TO THEM THEY LAUGH AND SAY TOMORROW ISN'T PROMISE AND THE DESTRUCTION CONTINUES ATTEMPTING TO USE YOUR ILLNESS AS A REASON TO CONTINUE THE WRONG THEY DO. IT SEEMS THAT THEY'RE TRYING TO TEMPT DEATH.

IF CANCER WINS I WILL ONLY BE UPSET BECAUSE I MAY NOT HAVE ACHIEVE THE GOALS I'VE SET FOR MYSELF AND MY FAMILY. BUT I WILL FIGHT CANCER AND ANY OBSTA-CLES TO ACHIEVE MY MISSION BECAUSE MY LIFE AND MY FAMILY DEPEND ON IT.

WARREN

THE ADVENTURE BEGINS

Before we look at where it starts, lets look at CANCER. CANCER is any of various malignant neoplasm characterized by the proliferation of anaplastic cells that tends to invade surrounding tissue and metastasize to new body sites. A pernicious spreading evil. MULTIPLE MYELOMA is a malignant proliferation of plasma cells in the bone marrow causing numerous tumors and characterized by the presence of an abnormal proteins in the blood.

Now where did cancer start? I don't think any one really knows. No one really started investigating until the start of the 20th Century. Doctor did notice that people were dying of some type of mysterious illness and there was nothing they could do. Some of the earlier cancers were from natural sources, which in their natural states were harmless, but when used in a concentrated form such as make-up the results were devastating. A lot of makeup in this country contained radioactive material. Women liked using the makeup because it would make them glow in the dark. Navy ships used radioactive indicators on doors and entrances so that they could be found in the dark. And in many areas cancer was result of high industrial area pollution.

In this modern age cancer has been linked to chemicals and new modern weapons. Cancers have been linked to Agent Orange, nuclear weapons, even some of the medicines being produced. I noticed that while I was in the hospital a lot of young soldiers were being treated for various forms of cancer. Then I notice in a documentary that some of our modern tanks are built with depleted Uranium a radioactive material. This makes me wonder. Sailors on nuclear ships working in the reactor area their children were born deformed. A coincidence I don't think so.

For me I believe my cancer started while I was at the Navy Inactive ships maintenance facility, Portsmouth Virginia. While there I was a team member on the radioactive material removal team. While there I didn't have any problems, but after I left my hair started to fall out, the navy doctor told me it was the shampoo. Next a bone in my right hand broke twice and all I got for that was a cast.

I finally started receiving treatment when doctors at Oaknoll Naval Hospital found that I had Multiple Myeloma. The process start when I complained of different problems and the doctors had me take a full physical. During this examination is when they found I had Cancer; next they gave me a series of other test including a bone marrow test (This test is where they took 3 pieces of bone out of your hip). Once they diagnosed me they started me on chemotherapy and that was in 1993. My life expectancy was less than 5 years. The severity of multiple myeloma is rated 1 to 4, with stage 4 being the most severe. I was a stage 4. Many of my fellow patients died within 2 years of being diagnosed. While being treated I was admitted to the Oaknoll Hospital several times for cancer related illnesses. The care by the Doctors and nurses was outstanding. What I liked was when they told me everything about my chemo. That was what it does and what effect it was having on me. With this positive attitude by the staff I didn't feel intimidated by any treatment. I was worried but not panic stricken.

When you think back on everything, all you can say is **WHAT A RIDE WHAT A RIDE.**

COPING

Having been diagnosed with Multiple Myeloma (bone cancer) almost four years ago, I was told by my doctor that the only thing I could look forward to would be years of Chemotherapy. For three years I was on the ride of my life. During that time, I was placed in several hospitals, Oaknoll Naval Hospital, Oakland California, Palo Alto V.A. Hospital, Palo Alto, California, Summitt Medical Center, Oakland California, and David Grant Medical Center, Travis Air Force Base, Fairfield California. I found myself being treated for high fevers; I had to have emergency surgery in my neck because a large blood clot had developed in a main vein. Next, I found I was allergic to plastic and all the lines that were used to administer Chemotherapy had to be removed. When I'm asked about this, I tell everyone that this is my greatest adventure, an adventure that could kill me, but an adventure still.

The VA Medical Center Puget Sound, Seattle, Washington notifies me that in a week I will be flown to Seattle, Washington for a bone marrow transplant. When I asked about a Donor, I was told that I would be my own donor. Immediately upon arrival in Seattle, the medical staff started testing my blood; to help my body produce more blood cells, daily I was given a substance call Growth Factor this was administered by needles in the stomach, next they gave me chemo. Thirty days later I was given intensive chemotherapy that lasted seven days. I was given thirty-five pills every six hours for three days, and for four days I was given liquid chemo through a Hickman catheter in my chest. My chemo consisted of Busulfan (sound like a coal by-product), Melphalan, and thiotepa all dangerous chemicals. Two days after completion of chemo the doctors started the transplant, this part lasted about a day. This is when the discomfort and misery actually start. ABOUT THE BONE MARROW TRANSPLANT-The transplant is where you are given intensive chemotherapy, which destroys the cancer, but it also destroys the bone marrow system, which produces your blood cells. The new blood cells donated by you or a donor are put into your blood system to restart your bone marrow system. Some patients also had to have radiation therapy in addition to the chemo; it depended on the type of cancer. Going through this process was painful and uncomfortable. For forty-five days I was fed food and water through IV tubes in my chest. Fourteen days after starting the process I was given morphine for about two weeks. I experienced nausea and diarrhea. The funniest thing that happened was when I fell out of bed, and knocked myself out, the next thing I remember were the nurses putting me back in bed. It was like a slow motion scene in the movies.

I experienced hallucinations and severe mucositis (your mouth, stomach, and throat fill with fluid) and pneumonia. The number of people that died in the course of this program surprised me. The fatality rate is at least 50 percent. Three patients died within the first two weeks of my being in the hospital. I wasn't worried about death though, because I felt that God had something special for me. When asked by Doctors what brought me this far, my answer was faith in God and belief in myself. Doctors asked me if I ever thought of committing suicide? I told them no because I was taught to have faith in God and to believe everything would be all right. Eating was hard to do because of nausea and diarrhea. It was a big accomplishment to eat a bowl of soup. I was kept on a liquid diet until I left the hospital, but by that time my liquid diet was reduced and I was eating some solid foods, not much but I was eating. I received three blood transfusions and I had to be readmitted to the ward for a GI track examination because of continual nausea due to mucositis.

Going though this Transplant is an experience you don't forget. The chemo destroys the lining of your mouth, throat and stomach. Your skin color changes, if you're black, you become blacker, if you're white you become darker. Your hair falls out, your immune system goes to zero which means you can't be around babies (because of the live vaccines used for immunization), pets, smoke, construction, crowds, buses, or anything that creates a fungus. You become so weak that walking a block or tying your shoes takes an effort.

My wife was with me for the duration of the program, sometimes spending the night with me in my room. As patients we had our support group, Once we were allowed to leave our room, we met in the outpatient room sometimes as a large group and sometimes it was just a couple of us. We discussed medicine treatments, different cancers, and the medical staff. Sometimes a doctor or nurse would talk to us and we could talk to them about any subject. My saddest experience was one patient named Scott; he talked to all of us and encouraged us. He had gone through treatments for five months and his body was rejecting all of the treatments. He came in every morning for treatment and blood transfusions; He would sit and talk with us while he was having his treatment. One morning he came into the outpatient's room in a wheel chair and told us good by. We thought he was going home, because he wanted to be with his two young sons; however he was told he had two weeks to live. He lived three weeks before his death. Now I'm told that Jim's transplant didn't take (his wife Jackie and my wife became close friends). He was released from the hospital a month ago and I've been informed that he was just put back in the hospital because he lost fifty lbs. since being sent home. Even after having the Transplant the shadow of cancer still hangs over you.

What did I think about while in the hospital? Well, for the first two or three weeks I didn't really think about much of anything. Knowing that other guys died shook me up, but that passed. I didn't worry about dying because of my belief that God didn't bring me this far to have me die in a hospital room. What re-enforced that attitude was the fact that most of the patients in the ward had been on chemo for less than one year and I had been taking chemo for the better part of three years. Every day was an adventure! Receiving fluids and liquid nutrition through a Hickman line in my chest was really an experience; I never felt hungry or thirsty, I still wanted the taste of a hamburger, tamale, fried chicken and seafood, but I wasn't hungry.

After about three weeks you were encouraged by the doctors and nurses to walk around the ward. I did that as often as possible. Sometimes I walked by myself; sometimes my wife or a nurse would walk with me. Sometimes I would use a wheelchair as a walker to move about the ward, and I would do this sometimes at 4:00 in the morning. It was great moving around because I could talk to people, I used the treadmill and the exercise bike. After five minutes on those I was exhausted, but I would go back and try them again and again. After six weeks I was given a one-day pass, then a 3-day pass. That was exciting because I could leave the hospital grounds but I still couldn't eat anything. The nurses started feeding me different soups to get me eating. There were some soups I could eat, but there were also some I couldn't. My wife made a soup for me that stayed down but the seasoning and spices she put in the soup had me hot and sweaty as if I were in 100-degree weather. But the soup tasted good, smile.

Even after leaving the room and being made an outpatient, I still had to adjust to eating and being around people. I had to adjust to nausea and using the toilet. I learned to adjust to everything because of great family support and because of support from the other outpatient and the nurses. When I got bored my wife, and my oldest son and I would play games my wife bought. Your family and friends outside of your little circle (the BMTU) haven't a clue, they assume it's almost business as usual, but any thing can set your schedule back. I wouldn't wish this experience on anyone. My wife and I were taught by the hospital staff to administer the liquid nutrition, fluids and medicine through the lines in my chest. We were also taught how to flush these lines to prevent clotting and infections. What did I think about this experience? I told my wife I was tired of being sick! After going through all this discomfort, pain and misery, you talk to people who are going through the program and two days after your conversation you find that they're dead! What type of foundation do you lean on? That's simple you put your faith in God and the belief that he hasn't brought you this far to let your soul be lost, but to save you and make you whole. A lot of people are afraid of chemo and the transplant, but I believe that I'm still here because of these treatments and early diagnosis (and support).

The BONE MARROW TRANSPLANT is a program that should be given more support by the Government and by the people. As a Black, I believe we should support the donor program. Is the bone marrow donor program painful or dangerous? The answer is no. The process is like a transfusion and is only required when needed. The problem is that there aren't enough black donors. To insure success in a transplant doctors try to get cells from the same racial group. A lot of us in the black community aren't familiar with the program. No one has really explained the need or the reason for the program; I think the government could do a better job of informing the general public about the bone marrow transplant. Some Blacks know about the donor program but they don't talk about it because they see cancer as a negative thing. Having Cancer is something none of us want, but once diagnosed we must think about family, income and treatment. Some suspect they may have cancer but refuse to see a Doctor and that's the big mistake because early diagnosis in many cases is the best cure. Insurance companies think of all types of reasons why they shouldn't treat you. Even the government tries to think of reasons why they shouldn't treat you; in many cases the government is the reason why we have this disease.

Because of the many Cancers being found, some of which are caused by radioactivity from government and civilian projects and some from various chemicals such as Agent Orange. We must be aware of the many diseases, prevention and cure and one of the most important cures is the BONE MARROW TRANSPLANT PROGRAM. We can help through the BONE MARROW DONOR PROGRAM. We must join in to combat this terrible disease known as Cancer.

For many of us, the BONE MARROW TRANSPLANT is our last stop, our last hope!

WHO PREPARED ME FOR THE TRANSPLANT?

Even though OakKnoll Naval Hospital administered my original chemotherapy. The responsibility of preparing me for the Bone Marrow Program goes to the VA clinic in Martinez, Ca. There I was under the care of the Hemo/Oncology department. The doctors responsible for me were DR O'Donnell and DR Edalman and their staff of doctors and nurses.

The staff at VA Martinez gave me the attention I needed to build up my body in preparation for the transplant; I was administered chemotherapy by nurses Karen and Pat. Rogg mixed chemo in the Pharmacy department, this also included steroids and if complications developed they had me admitted to David Grant hospital at Travis Air Force Base. After receiving all this attention and care they had built me up so much I looked like a professional football player. Through all the treatments they had very high spirits, even when I was placed in the hospital on numerous occasions for fevers and blood infections. The Staff's positive attitude has a lot to do with setting the tone for a patient, and for me it helped quite a lot.

Good Morning America

(I always wanted to say that)

First I want to give thanks to God for taking care of me and watching over me.

Now lets get down to business. Haven't you awakened in the morning, excited and enthusiastic about facing the day. Well, that's how I felt going into the Bone Marrow Transplant program. Doctors, nurses and counselors explained the ups and downs (I remember the downs), but the excitement was still there.

Once the transplant started and I was taken off morphine, I would work my way to the radio (every room was provided a CD/cassette player/w radio and a television) and turn to some R & B and have my own jam session. When the doctors came to check on me in the morning they would turn the radio down, when they left my room I would turn the volume back up. I enjoyed my time in the hospital, but like everyone else I was anxious to leave. All through my cancer treatment I received support from family and friends. I received a lot of support and encouragement from my doctors and nurses. This support is sometimes more important than medicine. Your strongest support is from family and friends. A friendly hello from family and friends is worth a thousand words. Doctors and Nurses can only do so much, so the rest of your support has to come from outside. You need someone willing to talk, to laugh, joke and watch television with you. You need someone who is really able and willing to share those up and down moments. That's what I consider support.

ALL OF US PATIENTS PUT OUR

ALL INTO THE PROGRAM. WE MET

MANY SUCCESS AND MANY FAILURES.

SOME DIED BUT WE ALL CONSIDER

OURSELVES WINNERS.

The thing about the transplant process and all the medication is that it works on you physically and mentally. The mental part I would deal with by playing cribbage and yahtze and talking to my son Damien and his family. Damien took many days off from his job to spend time with me. And there was my friend Gene who flew from Oakland to visit me. For the physical I would walk the ward. After being in bed for so long walking became a new experience. You felt like a baby learning to walk. Many times my wife or a nurse assisted me. If they weren't available I would use a wheel chair as a walker. It was exciting to finally be able to use the treadmill. When I was finally able to get around without assistance I did a little jig, it was nice to be mobile.

RECOVERY!

Recovery where does it start? Your recovery starts officially on the day you leave the hospital to go home because the complete time you're assigned to the hospital you're under observation for infections or your body's rejection of the cells donated to you. I found out that if you have any additional medical problems the intense chemo might even attack that problem. One patient required surgery on his leg due to some type of blood infection, another had to have surgery on her chest because of a hole in her lung. Another had to wear an oxygen bottle after starting the program. One of the guys that died during the course of the program, we were told that his being overweight was one of the contributing factors.

With all the discomfort I went through in the hospital my wife and I were part of a medical team along with the doctors, nurses, chaplain, psychologist and social worker and our assignment was to get me through this medical procedure with as few problems as possible (hopefully none) and we succeeded. I don't believe I would be here today if they hadn't been there to help. When the team started that was when my recovery started.

After about 2 months I was allowed to go to the apartment provided to me and my family by the hospital. Staying at the apartment meant I had to start adjusting to regular life. And this is a learning experience. Having been taught how to use the IV lines in my chest my wife and I had to start using that training at the apartment to administer liquid nutrition and medicine. Taking liquid nutrition was a 12 to 14 hour process and sometimes longer if you had to stop and administer antibiotics (this was if you only had the use of one pump). With all this fluid going in when did it all come out? Well, the answer is every hour! That's right every hour, you had to go to the bathroom.

Now what about eating? That was the hardest part to adjust to because anything you ate would come back up. You would start with soups, fruit, next meats and solid foods. To me it was mind over matter. I was encouraged by the doctors to keep trying. I seemed to make some progress so the doctors reduced my liquid nutrition intake. Once my stomach rejected all food and liquid; I couldn't eat or drink anything for 2 days. Any attempt to try and eat would result in the food coming up. So it was back to 100% liquid nutrition. What did I think about this experience? I told my wife I was tired of being sick! We didn't have a car so we rode back and forth to the hospital with other patients, sometimes we rode the bus. We went to downtown Seattle, to the movies, museum, Pikes Place and the amusement park. All this was exciting but tiring. Walking up a hill was like running 10 miles. Some of the other patients (these patients were further along in the program than I) encouraged me to go out and do things; they even took us out to dinner a few times.

During all this time the Doctors and Nurses saw me daily and they encouraged me all the time. During these visits to see the Doctors I was given medication to help me eat better and antibiotics to fight any infections. My blood was tested daily and for one series of tests the nurses took twenty tubes of blood, I was also given 3 blood transfusions.

Now that I'm home I find things to keep me busy. There are a lot of things I can't do, but I still manage to keep busy. The recovery lasts about 2 years which means you're under doctors observation during that time. This means blood test weekly (2 to 3 times a week in the beginning), x-rays, MRI examination and the list goes on. If you have a problem the doctors check it immediately. The nurses whether here at the Clinic in Martinez, Ca. or at the Va. Medical Center in Seattle, Washington will answer any question.

After being home 4 months I'm doing better. I have occasional diarrhea, nausea, aches and pains, which come and go quickly. I see my doctor once a week. My medicines consist of vitamins and mineral and a couple of medicines for my immune system. I feel blessed, because a lot of my fellow patients aren't doing as well. You become like a family, so these things upset you, but you continue to push on.

I've found that going though recovery is not just medical, but also a mental and physical exercise. Since being home the electricity was turned off in our place because we hadn't paid the electrical bill. I thought my wife had paid the bill and she thought I had paid the bill. After checking with the P.G. & E., I found that my bill was going to Seattle Washington. I had to pay the bill plus $200.00 (as a security deposit) to have the lights turned on.

Next, I had to take my truck into the shop because I was hearing a loud noise in the front end. After checking, the dealer told me the brakes were gone on the front wheels. I couldn't understand this because my truck was only nine months old when I was admitted to the hospital. The dealership said apparently someone had dogged my truck while I was in the hospital; the repair bill was $400.00. I can't afford to pay these types of expenses they're non-productive and they put a strain on you mentally and financially especial when you're trying to recover.

I've lost 50 pounds, but my weight has been stable for a month. Next is the mental and physical fatigue and to combat this you must have a positive I can do attitude. I'm not complaining but I am looking at the problems and obstacles that confront me and what I must do to navigate a positive course of action. One thing I've learned is that first you must recognize a problem whether it's yourself, someone or something. Next you work to solve it. The sad thing about being positive, is people question your being ill because they think you're suppose to be looking frail and all cut up from operations.

Now I'm home dealing with the people out here in the real world. People think that you should sit back and enjoy your disability check. They want you to volunteer your services. To all this I say no. To me it's a black thing, if you want me; show me some cash. As a black contractor before going in the Hospital I couldn't get any real support for my business. Everyone had a negative answer for everything from finance to paperwork. Now that I'm home and striving to recover everyone is thinking of all types of reason why I should do things voluntarily. If you say no than they want to question your motives. While going through recovery I still try to improve my business. Why do I stay in business? I believe I can beat the opposition and at 54 years old I've got plenty of time.

I Wonder

Having cancer and going through recovery gives me a lot of time to think and imagine. I wonder about all sorts of things, my illness, family, and friends. I think of where I would like to be, and the goals I've set for myself and life in general. I also think about that vacation I always wanted to take.

I see new businesses on the stock market and wonder why my business isn't there. Many times I tell myself I understand why I'm not there. But, I still get upset, because I wonder if I was given true opportunity, training, and support early in life things may have been different. My brother-in-law once told me that I don't get real support, because to a lot of people I look too proud and I'm knowledgeable on what I am talking about. Because I don't get that all needed support, I wonder if what he says is true. I'm knowledgeable about many things, but that's because I've been taught about a variety of subjects, plus I've experienced quite a lot during my travels around the globe. When I was in the Navy, I was an electrician in engineering. There you're taught to be problem solvers. Being confined to those windowless vessels sometimes for long periods of time took management, leadership and business skills. What kept those ships running was us sailors, working our magic through our imagination using skills learned through on the job training and the various schools that the military had us attend.

Being out and in a different work environment is really something. I already understood that there would be adjustments, but, your thinking also changes (the way in which you think). A lot of the electrical and electronic experience I gained has been lost due to non-use. I'm not able to put many of the skills acquired during my military career to use. I wonder what may have happened if some of the work on ships that was turned over to civilians had been picked up by us retired military personnel who are now businessman. Some of us see our retirement as a way to make use of our skills in the way we want. I WONDER!

Have you sometimes wondered why you're so eager to spend your money especially when you see something on sale. Buying something you don't even need, Instead of taking that money and investing. Many times I read in the paper of people who became millionaires in what appeared to be overnight. Most of the people didn't become millionaires overnight; many took their money and over a long period of time invested instead of continually spending.

Have you ever wondered about Stock Market? It has been around quite sometime. Many of us Blacks haven't been encouraged to utilize it. Seeing it as a playground for whites. Not realizing that fortunes are made and lost there.

I watch those spacecraft go into space and it's always someone white at the controls. Yes, there are blacks in the space program, but when it comes to television you always see Whites, Japanese, Russians, and Frenchman. Where are the Blacks or Africans? I believe that the Propulsion Plant of the future will be created by someone of color. These things I don't wonder about because time I believe will prove me correct. I wonder if upon completion of treatment will I be allowed to utilize my skills the way I want and use those skills profitably. I wonder will my future be bright or will everyone attempt to steer my future differently.

I wonder about many things, life, death, hope and faith. I don't dwell on the things I wonder about, but I use them in my decision making because they help me move ideas around. One of my neighbor call it reflecting because to him you're looking back on the past and the decisions we made that affected our future. But to me it also means you're curious about what's on the other side of the street.

Here in America were opportunity is suppose to be available for everyone for many black Americans true opportunity is held back or just plain denied. Opportunity denied or held back by blacks and whites, but controlled by whites. Blacks have been part of the American system for three hundred years, free from slavery for over one hundred. I have one question where is our glory. Japan was devastated by two atomic bombs; Korea was destroyed by war and conflict. In the pass fifty years many of those countries that were poor, enslaved and part of the colonial system have shown fantastic growth and influence in the world financially and politically. What has happened to blacks in America? We have no major corporations that have any influence or impact, but it appears every one is trying to control our lives. Politically we have some, but very little influence. I've always felt that I was missing something. It appear that everything was passing me by, I was going only so high, moving only so far, going only so fast. As one of my customers told me we black have been missing out on many things because of inhibitions we've been taught. Something has always been left out. What has been left out? There is a long list. I can think of many things where we blacks have been left out of the picture. Examples: Health, life, death, money, and advancement. With education and technology we're always behind always being introduced to new ideas after the fact, never really being a visible part of change. We have always been taught to work for someone, for something to be successful someone white must be charge. As time passes we find that these things aren't true, because of the lack of proper education life has taken its toll on many of us.

What would happen if we were allowed true economical, and political freedom? What would happen if we took charge and stop that old teaching of questioning our ability? What if we stop blaming ourselves for many of our social problems and place the blame where it belongs. I WONDER!

When I'm facing a problem wondering help me focus on a solution. When you wonder it helps you decide on other paths for a solution because you become curious and say what if. Going into the transplant program was a what if situation. When I spoke to the program director he told me I could die. When I asked if they had any type of success record to go on I was told no. But I still said yes. As I go through recovery I find that what the doctor says is true they have a very poor success record for the Bone Marrow Transplant but for many of us its our last hope so we must take that great leap of faith. Of the 13 that went through the program with me only 5 of us survive. The most recent casualty was Jim Collier his transplant fail and he died after a 2-year struggle. Why do we fight so hard, especially when confronting such terrible odds? We have that desire to win. Have you wanted to do something but didn't and wondered what would happen if you did. The next time you have an idea don't sit on it or worry about the inhibitions or dangers you've been taught, try it the results may surprise you

SNOOPY, WELCOME HOME

Tom and I wish you greetings from Oregon. Tom is the Son-in-law of my friend Jim. The weather is sunny, but here in the Portland Oregon area it

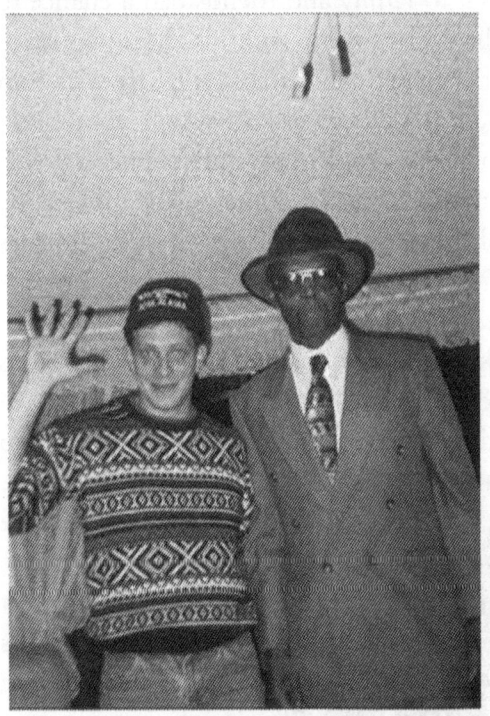

is always attempting to rain, occasionally there are snow flurries. Everyone talks about the rain in Seattle, but I don't think they have been to Portland. The sun is now pushing its ways through the clouds letting the heat from its rays warm your body. Today was a very nice day for a memorial service. At the church where the service was held, everyone gathered old friends, and new friends every-one hugged, embraced or just shook hands. Flowers were everywhere and the Bagpiper walked through playing his instrument. Although this was a memorial for someone special who had left this world to many of us this was a pleasant time.

Today was the memorial service for Jim Collier (Special Forces name Snoopy) a fellow Bone Marrow Transplant patient. Jims transplant failed, but he continued to fight physically, mentally, and spiritually. Spiritually was the most important because his faith in God helped him to endure the pain and discomfort. On the day of his death he died smiling and many of us believe this is because the first thing God said to Jim was **WELCOME HOME.**

At his memorial service he was honored by a color guard made up of members of the local Vietnam Veterans Organization. There were even members from his old Special Operations unit. During the memorial service everyone from his minister, to family and friends had a chance to speak. Many got up and talk of their relationship with Jim. Many spoke of his service time where in combat they felt comfortable and safe with him because he was always someone who would always watch your back. During his illness here was a man who took time out to interact with everyone. He was in the church chorus, a regular at the weekly bible study he served as chaplain for the local Vietnam Veterans organization. Jim was a man who through out his lifetime reached out and touched everyone, crossing all social and ethnic lines. As a fellow cancer patient I found that here was a man that I could talk to, someone willing to listen. As I was going through the Bone Marrow Transplant, I remember my inability to eat, the desire was there but nothing would stay down. Encouraging me to

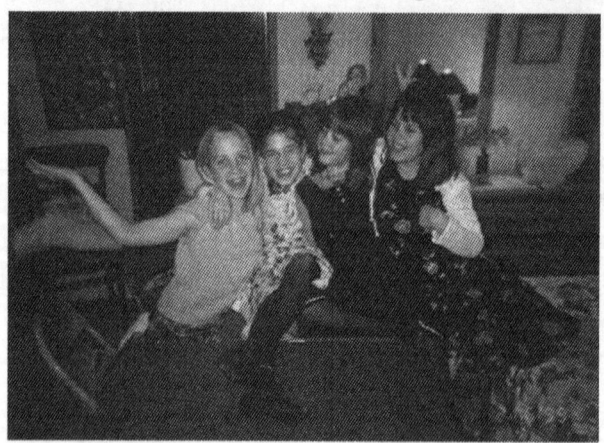

eat Jim and his wife Jackie would take me and my wife Frances out to dinner. Now as I walk through his house from room to room getting to know how Jim was, I smile. I remember Jim sitting in the hospital outpatient room waiting to start his transplant and after starting his transplant visiting him in his room, and always with him whether in the apartment provided by the hospital or in his hospital room was his wife Jackie. Although I left the hospital before him, he would still call or send E-mail over the computer and we would compare notes. Now I hear his grandchildren playing in the next room, sometimes they would come out and give me hugs and kisses. His children are going through the rooms sorting out all of Jims belongings. I looked through his pictures from high school to present seeing him grow, having a family, and though all the travel of military service taking time out to help his daughters celebrate their first birthday, taking his family to Germany and after getting out of the service taking his wife to Hawaii celebrating their 25th anniversary.

Lets not forget his military service time where after serving in Germany he was transferred to Vietnam, Cambodia, and Thailand where saw combat. During his service time he received many metals and commendations including the bronze star. Here was a man who served with the Army Special Forces having served in Special operations for the government. A man who never stopped thinking of family and no matter what the job or situation kept his faith in God and he always supported the military.

Looking in his office I see his computer, this he used to keep in contact with all his friends. There is his laptop computer for keeping notes sitting on the floor. Looking in a corner I see his stereo with the old 8 track player and record player. On the wall hangs his collection of military awards, plaques and flays from his old combat units. Even with all this there was stillroom for his grand-children's toys. Now his office is slowly being disassembled and sent everywhere.

In the living room many of us gather as we talk about Jim and how he became the person we learn to know. Over on the love seat is his mother and mother-in-law with his sister standing near-by. And on the sofa is a fellow serviceman and veteran. For many of us this is a sad moment because another comrade has fallen to cancer. But, his memories will always be with us and we can have comfort and joy in knowing he is now with God.

Remembrance

All things work together for good to them who love the Lord. Romans 8: 28

PEACE

A Lighter Side: Food to Eat, Things to Do, Places to See

What do you do after all those down periods? Well, you don't dwell on them! That's a good way to hurt yourself. Find something to do or a place to go. It's great being out of the hospital and off liquid nutrient and that regular liquid diet. With Liquid nutrient I was fed through an IV tube in my chest, I couldn't eat anything except when the hospital was preparing to release me. A liquid diet is where your food is in a liquid form (Jell-O, Soup, and Tea) with no seasoning. The stuff is terrible and quite bland. Now that I can eat everything, what do I want? Lets start with some Greens (collards, mustard greens, and kale), seasoned with a nice tender ham hock. Don't forget to throw in some new potatoes. Or how about some fresh green beans just picked. For meat how about some fresh ham or some tender fried chicken cooked in real fat. A nice piece of tender lamb cooked and seasoned the Greek way on a grill accompanied by stuffed grape leaves and a salad of lettuce, tomatoes, Kalamada olives, and feta cheese covered with seasoned olive oil. After eating relax with some pastry and Greek espresso coffee.

Too hot to cook indoors; how about a Bar-B-Que? Get that fire going and Que some Ribs and chicken covered in that special sauce; and the sauce has to be spicy. Don't forget those Hot Links. Serve everything with some baked beans and potato salad. While I'm waiting for the food to cook relax with some fresh watermelon and sip a nice cool soda. And for

Seafood I like Blue crabs, fried flounder, fresh fried shrimp and fried oysters. And my wife's Gumbo with its shrimp, crab, sausage, okra and seasoned to perfection.

I'm making myself hungry, I think I'll ask my wife to light the Grill(smile).

To the Beach

My wife and my sister-in-law says off to the beach we go. All of us including my nephew, niece and the grand kids jump in the van and were off to the beach. To Santa Cruz we go for a day of sun and catching that cool breeze off the surf. Although Santa Cruz is a busy amusement area we found a parking spot with no problem. Then everyone rushed inside to enjoy the rides. There were plenty of rides for everyone and the smaller kids. There was Roller Coaster, bumper cars and plenty of rides for the small kids. My youngest grandson favorite ride was the Big Rig Convoy he rode that about five times. The older kids rode on every ride they could. We walked the full length of the board walk. Afterward we walked out on to the pier. This is where the restaurants are located. Instead of going inside of a restaurant we ordered our lunch and sat out front and caught the summer breeze. We stop to see the Mary Wilson Show (formerly of the Supremes) and it was very good. Don't forget the sandy beach! The kids played and splashed in the water. We finally returned home about 11pm. Everyone enjoyed themselves.

You don't want to go to the beach? How does a fashion show sound? You say no, not a fashion show what does that have to do with cancer. To recover you must encourage yourself to get back into circulation and socialize with people; Socializing stimulates your thinking. In the building where I live one of the artist had an open studio. Artist have open studio exhibits to allow people to become familiar with their work. In the building where I live in we have a lot of artist, there are also engineers, computer programers many with their own businesses. The feature artist was Jill Banashek ,artist and writer. It was a nice exhibit with plenty of food, wine and entertainment. There was a very nice crowd .One of the main attraction was Salsa lessons by Gabriel Romero and Alicia Chacon. They were performing at Kimballs a popular gathering night spot in Emeryville, California. The lessons and performance was outstanding. When it was time for everyone to participate in the lesson no-one held back. If you had 2 left feet no-one notice. Everything was nice the art exhibit and the lessons. You must remember that its not just your physical self that must recover, but also your mental self. In my effort to get around and find things to I've found that there is always something to do. Remember, you want to be better now than what you were when the illness and treatment started. Don't sit and mope, look and you will find there are plenty of things to keep you busy. These are things you want to do, not what other people want. I've found that people are always trying to maneuver you. They have no consideration for the things you're concerned about. You must gently ease them to the side and you work on your needs and ideas. Don't worry they will understand and work with you. People will have to understand that even though you have cancer you still have desires and goals and you know your limitations.

When I was in High School I wrote myself this poem which was later printed in the school newspaper.

IT NEVER PAYS TO SIT AND STARE FOR YOU WILL NEVER GET ANYWHERE, SO GET UP OFF YOUR SEAT RIGHT NOW AND MOVE YOUR LAZY SOUL AROUND.

I still remember that poem today and it's true, so do something.

WHAT DO I THINK ABOUT ALL THIS?

What do I think about this complete thing? Well it's an experience you don't forget. From diagnoses to chemotherapy to time in the hospital to transplant to recovery its all something I wouldn't want to repeat or wish on anyone. Through all this I felt like a building that had been set ablaze and chemo and all the medical treatment was there to stop the blaze progress. And the increased dosage of Chemo was shoring put in place to keep me from collapsing.

My first chemo was a hand full of pills I had to take for four days a month. Next the chemo was changed to the IV type which was stronger. This stuff was so toxic that it would kill a healthy person. At home I had to have a bio-hazard kit because I couldn't allow these chemicals to touch my skin. It was pumped into me 24hrs a day, 4 days a month even when I slept I could hear the pump. It felt as if someone was always beating on me. I felt weak and tired, I slept a lot and until I finally adjusted I had to sit even to use the toilet.

The Bone Marrow Program is the same as remodeling a building. You receive intensive Chemotherapy and if necessary Radiation therapy which is needed to destroy all infectious cancer material, it changes you inside and out. The Bone Marrow Transplant is a scary procedure. Unlike surgery where they remove the cancer by cutting it out, after the removal of the cancer many times you can feel comfortable because its removal is immediate. But with the Bone marrow Transplant nothing is immediate because it destroys your Bone Marrow system which produces your red blood cells, and it also destroys your immune system. The new transplant cells you're given are the new building blocks. For ten days after administration of your new cells you are under close observation by doctors and nurses to insure your body is beginning to recover. Next you're given antibiotics, steroids and a host of medicines to get you though, a lot about your survival depends on you mentally and your diet because there are foods that can help you. And don't drink or smoke because this can counter the effect of the drugs and medicines you're taking. And don't believe that thing about marijuana helping you. Sure it helps with pain when dealing some cancers but it has a fungus that can be hazardous to transplant patient. How do I know I ask my doctors about it and they sat an explained the pros and cons and one of my fellow patients tried it and he ended up in worse trouble health wise.

It's Getting Tough, But You Must Be Tougher

How are you feeling? Recently I passed out in the Clinic due to a sinus infection. A few weeks later I had to be admitted to the hospital for 4 days due to internal bleeding. I had to go to the hospital twice. Once for a fever and the second time for something they call vertigo. With vertigo the room appears to be always spinning around and you walk as if you're intoxicated. I stayed at the hospital 4 hrs. Even with things getting tougher mentally, I still feel great. Now I must go to the Clinic for a check-up because I've had a tingling in my back. The tingling runs from the base of my neck to my legs. I feel this tingling when I bend my head down or change positions of my arm. It's not uncomfortable when you're sitting even though you're aware of what's happening. When walking. it causes you to pause for a while (to stand still). I still can't run because my feet have a spongy feel at times, but I think that can be corrected with a change of shoes. If I try to run I feel as if I'm a hundred years old. There is a name for all this activity but I can't pronounce it.

There have been all types of x-rays taken of my head, neck and spine; I'm told everything is fine, but sometimes I wonder. I felt this lump at the bottom of my rib cage it was checked and found to be just bone. I feel a little uncomfortable because the Cancer doctors at the clinic are really overworked. Sometimes I wonder if I would get better treatment at another hospital. With all the cut backs you have to believe that you're getting the best with what's available, or are we? My regular doctor is out with pneumonia and his partner is overworked.

I didn't see the neurologist today because no one could find my medical chart. This is the third time this has happened and I feel uncomfortable about it. I don't really like the neurologist because they appear to be impersonal and it seems that they trivialize my situation. I don't expect them to be jumping up and down, but something is missing. For a lot of us patients the doctors are our line of defense and their success is based on our success. As long as my records were kept in the hematology/oncology department they were not lost or misplaced, now they're floating around in space somewhere. This annoys me since all of my medical information is in those records.

My weight is stable. I had dropped from 218 lbs. to 168 lbs. my weight has now stabilized at 186 lbs. Losing that weight bothers me because I was down to skin and bone, very little muscle. Losing that weight was unnerving because when I looked at my legs they look like tooth picks. I try to lift things to buildup my muscles but, there are something's I just can't move without help. People look at me strangely because as a cancer patient I'm always attempting to do things, they still think you're supposed to look sickly. I still tire easily, the heat still kicks my butt , however, my appetite has really improved since they cured my sinus infection.

THE NORM

What is the NORM-This is what society considers normal. There are a lot of things that are normal or the norm. But I want to talk about the things that aren't normal, things that are taught to us. People with cancer all die, we're all bigots and racists. All these statements are false. These are thoughts we're all taught from childhood.

Everyone with Cancer does not die. Many of us don't go around looking sickly, many of us aren't cut-up from operations and our hair is still there just thinner. Because of new treatments, a change of diet and lifestyle, many of us don't die. We still have aches and pains, but we work to survive. The thing that bothers me is that if I don't appear sickly then people and doctors tend to not take my illness seriously.

Bigotry and Racism are taught to us from birth and unknowingly we except this as normal. These attitudes must change because they're constantly affecting all our daily lives.

RESPONSIBILITY

Have you wondered about the terms-Assistance and Help. There is a big differences. I tell my wife to quit trying to help everyone, you can assist people but don't help. When you help people many becoming dependent on you. And if possible they will shift part of their responsibility to you making you accountable for their action. And the complete time they receive your help their position on many things never change. When they fall you pick them up, when they have a problem they expect you to solve it. There is no accountability when things go wrong because everything has been put on your shoulders. They can be relatives, friends or associates. Many times when things go wrong they make you feel that you're partly or fully responsible and that you should repair the problem. In other words they want you to agree to the wrong that they're doing, so watch it when helping people. Don't stop helping people but realize that there is a cut-off point. Sometimes you must remember you're only one person and you can't solve everybody's problems especially when they don't want to help themselves.

When you give people assistants this means that in many cases they're already out there trying to do something. The assistant may be financial, transportation, a telephone or even an office and roof over their head. They don't want to be dependent on you or anyone else. They have dreams and they're trying to make that dream work. Myself, I ask for assistant from banks, friends and relative and many act as if I'm begging. How can I be begging when I'm working with my own tools, my imagination and what funds I have available to achieve my goals. You run into a problem and no-one really wants to answer your questions or assist you in dealing with it. Sometimes you know the solution but you understand that solving the problem takes more than yourself. I try to make it clear that I'm not begging I'm seeking assistants.

What this all leads up to is responsibility. Some of us want to be responsible, to take hold of our future and make things work. We take a project and strive to make it work. Given a problem we solve it. People look at us as foolish because they think that if you wait the problem will solve itself, sure it will but not always the way you want. There are a lot of people who want the benefits but not the responsibility. They believe it's always someone else responsibility to take care of them. As long as something is free they will go along with the program even when they know the outcome. Being responsible you see the objectives, weigh the possible results and go to work, if things don't work out the way you want than you go back over things find the problem, make corrections and start again. Haven't you notice how some people will see a problem and their first responds is don't worry some one will fix it. No-one wants to be responsible. The end result can be catastrophic. In fighting the cancer that has attempted to take control of my body I have to take responsibility physically, spiritually, and mentally of myself and my future to win. And it's going to be a fight. Even with this I say.

PEACE MAY WE ALL PROSPER

THIS IS A GROWING EXPERIENCE

Going through recovery and attempting to rebuild yourself is a growing and learning experience. You learn to draw on all the positive things you were taught from childhood to adulthood. You find that it is so easy to dwell on those negative thoughts, things that can hinder or slow your recovery, and it takes will power to draw on those positive things. You learn that many times you not only have to face your fears, but you must also confront others attitudes because they will attempt to give you reason to fail in any endeavor. I find that to recover I must draw on those things taught or shown by example.

Believing In Yourself

Having come to California from Virginia 11 years ago, I've found that I've faced more hostility and harassment now than at anytime in my life; both as a business owner and a black laborer. This harassment comes from blacks, whites, family and friends. People try to dictate to you what you should do, yet have no intention of assisting you, their only intention is to get as much out of you as possible (time and money).

I started my business here in 1990 with the tools I had and my last paycheck. Business picked up so I hired my sons, another electrician, a receptionist and my wife. As business improved many people, including relatives said I was selfish and were continually saying what I should be doing for them. I tried to get the family to invest in my business but to no avail. The idea of me being selfish I couldn't understand; I was paying everyone a regular pay check and tried to involve them in my plans. I had projects that I didn't make money, yet I still paid everyone on time. Due to inexperience in estimating I seriously underbid on two apartment complexes (separate jobs), one my pay and profit totaled one dollar and the other project I didn't make anything, but I made sure everyone else was paid and that included relatives.

I offered people fantastic deals and guaranteed the price on all projects, yet we were mostly shunned on a lot of them. One black contractor told me that he had heard of us and that we had an excellent reputation, but he could get people on drugs to perform the work a lot cheaper. One of my relatives was building a two unit building which failed 2 city inspections I offered to finish the electric phase of the building; his cost would only be to pay my helper. Instead he hired an inexperienced and alcoholic laborer, the building failed again. I had to step in at my own expense and use my sons to finish the work.

As a Black who has seen many changes, I find that many times people don't take us serious and that include many Blacks. Why has my business not grown? It's because of lack of real support. That in time of crisis everyone is really trying to think of reason why the business should fail. People say they want you to succeed but their actions show they want you to fail. Are they afraid of your success especially when your success benefits everyone? As a Businessman I've learn that in operating your business you have to be everything, owner, manager, marketer, labor, and finance manage, but as a Black businessman many want to view you as laborer. And for your business to be successful and grow you can't have yourself view as labor, but owner and organizer. When we Blacks attempt to rise above the labor label that is when the problem starts. It's as if people feel that we know too much or we want too much. Banks and financial institutes find reason not to deal with us. Legislator find loopholes in the law to circumvent us, many Blacks fine reasons not to deal with us preferring to go to other social groups. To me the situation is unnerving.

After completing the transplant and coming home from the Hospital I was really surprised to find my place and the shop changed around. Some of my office equipment was removed; in the shop things were rearranged (taken off the shelves) and stacked on shelves in the center. Some changes I could understand, but I felt that everyone had written me off believing I wouldn't recuperate. You learn to understand that people don't have the faith you do.

HEROES

We all need some type of heroes. To some of us our number one Hero is Jesus Christ. Sometimes people forget that a hero doesn't always fight the system; many times he or she struggles within the system to make it work. That's what I believe Dr. King was trying to teach.

You have people like Heavyweight Champ George Foreman who as the oldest Champion fought tremendous odds to regain the title. Next, there is Johnny Cochran the Black attorney that defended O.J. Simpson. He fought tremendous odds to win his case especially when many (mostly Whites and some Blacks) were saying Simpson was guilty. These are people that inspire us when things look tough. And there is also Dr C. Dianne Howell owner of the Black Business Listing who has always encouraged me.

My father, a writer in Washington, D.C. and fluent in 3 languages talked and counseled me all the time (he's seventy-six years old) he and I still talk on the phone frequently. My grandfather the son of slaves, had only a third grade education but he built one of the largest farms in the Black community of Hilltop, Maryland; he also became a master carpenter. With all this he supported a family of fourteen

With all this positive energy flowing, you try to draw on every-thing. Of course, I've had my ups and downs; with the recovery you draw on everything. There are a lot of foods you can't eat you become exhausted easily. After doing two hours of any work I have to lay down and sleep, I can't drink carbonated sodas because my muscles all over start to cramp, my body does not make a lot of saliva which means I can't eat any dry type foods. If I get up too fast I get light headed with the possibility of passing out. If I stand in the heat or sun too long it's almost instant that I become exhausted. I have battles with all types of problems, some I win and some I lose, but I say this time I say victory will be mine.

DESTINED TO FAIL

Here in America blacks are taught to under achieve, to accept things as they are, and not to question. With this line of thinking we are allowing people to always consider us underachiever, with this type of thinking we now encourage people to view Black civil rights as a nuisance instead of an issue. If we accept this line we as a social group are destine to fail never reaching our full potential.

We perform well as athletes, and as entertainers and you will find us in every segment of daily life reaching for greater heights but where is our victory. We have been taught that we will only go so high and we are taught that this is because of our mental and physical inability. Through many avenues this thinking is encouraged and this train of thought is based on images and stories created during slavery and later amplified to justify the positions create for us. Some very good examples of encouraging you to underachieve is the recent incident where a black man was dragged to death by 3 whites in Texas. Another is where a white youth shoots a Black because he felt the black didn't belong in the neighborhood. In New York, City four white policemen shot an unarmed Black merchant 19 times. Now how many times can you kill a person? And a very recent incident was recorded in Independence, Virginia where 2 whites were convicted of beheading a Black man. In Warren, Ohio to cover-up his attempted suicide a white priest claimed 2 Black men assaulted him and in San Diego, California a Black marine was crippled after being beaten and kicked by five whites. These aren't incidents that are brought on by criminal activity, But by the racial hate taught and consented to by the American society. With incidents such as these people are hesitant to achieve finding comfort hiding in the shadows. More and more blacks talk of prison as an honorable institution forgetting that the rights and privileges they complain about not having are automatic lost when convicted of certain crimes. Drugs use is on the rise. Sure drugs have been used for many years but never to the extent of today. People may laugh about the use of drugs but look around, you complain about cigarettes but you turn your back to hard drug use that is another form of slavery, a destroyer of souls, and a destroyer of family.

Many times through the media there is created a Black male/female atmosphere of distrust were we question each other's ability or position. We are even taught to question our decision-making ability. These are things that eventually lead to a weakening of the Black family structure. Accepting these things we allow ourselves to underachieve always continuing to accept all failures as normal. In politics we vote in a president and every effort is made to remove him from office. Why or how this happen no one really knows, but for many blacks confronted continually with race hate, these incident are examples of how far people will go with their hate to stop you from performing or achieving.

You are taught to be good in athletics, but there is little or no real training in executive skills. You're taught technical skills, but nothing about really using true creative skills and foresight. If you accumulate wealth, you're criticized for not giving it away. Even in politics limitations are placed on you and in many instances a negative image is create. The average life span of something black is about 10 years, many large businesses fade away, politicians going longer but much of the clout diminishes. No one is taught to look into the future and imagine what may happen or changes that may occur.

Many Blacks are taught to fear success or the accumulation of wealth in fear that it will upset Whites. Some Blacks today are being taught by their parents and the church that they shouldn't try to rise too high or too fast and they shouldn't accumulate a lot of money or property. If you do, you are made to feel you are some type of criminal, and you are taught to be suspicious of those who do. Don't complain about anything because many would see you as a threat, and attempt to either intimidate you or throw you to the dogs (this included both Blacks and Whites). Blacks will state that they will help you, but when the going gets tough they say the man (Whites) will hurt you, so they leave you out there by yourself. I was with a group of Black contractors and our complaint was how we as contractor were being treated. We decided to take out a full-page advertisement in one of the local Black newspapers to let the public know we were out there and what our position was on local contracts. We all agreed to pay $500.00 each for the advertisement, several days before the article was to be printed most of the contractors backed out because no-one wanted their pictures printed. Their reason was that if the white contractors saw their pictures they wouldn't give them any work. My answer was their seeing us was the least of our worries because most white contractor on large public projects contracted very little if any work to Blacks. After a 2-hour debate we agreed to print the article. A week later when I saw the article there was no pictures or any mention of any of us that paid for the advertisement. It looks like the one's that feared the whites got their way. It's amazing how many won't give us Black contractors large contracts or loans, but, everyone can tell us why we fail.

Sure we attend the same school system as everyone, but our educational training is considered below the national average. Everyone is saying that we should encourage our kids to use computer, but to use computers kids have to know how to read and speak. When we ask for funding for better education and training, we're told there is no funding available. But the government is always anxious to spend billions sending our youth to fight wars in foreign countries. If you do well in education you're treated as though something is wrong because you've set yourself apart from what is considered the norm. If you perform well on the job you told that it's because you got assistance from some social program, credit is never given to your ability.

Many White's are encouraging this line of thinking and that is why we rise only to certain levels, that is why there are no black C. E. O. 's in large national corporations, and very few of us in any positions of high political influence. As a cancer patient I've been able to have a successful recovery because I refuse to accept those images and attitudes of having low expectations because if I do I'm DESTINE TO FAIL.

FIGHTING NEGATIVE THINKING

I hate being sick because it gives people reason not to use you. Sure people will sit and talk to you, but many times I believe that they are just listening to please you. Sure I want people to listen, because I'm still full of ideas, but many people still talk about why you shouldn't or can't. As a Black man I've become tired of people always telling me or suggesting that I should work for someone else. When we say no then they begin thinking of reasons why things can't be done. I believe people have allowed themselves to be taught to fear us mainly for political and economical gain. Why I don't know because we only make up about 10–15% of the American population. It seems that every time people talk about Black issues it's always made to appear that everything is our fault or that we taught ourselves to think the way we do. People are so quick to forget that we as a people were taught and many times encouraged to act and think the way we do and when we attempt to be different we're put in a corner and ignore. I ask this question? As a group other than blacks have you done anything for us? Some individuals have made important efforts in assisting us. But what is needed is a positive productive change in society. Many whites resist that change why because they control the economic structure. Many people still see whites as the master and Blacks as the slave or servant and when speaking to us it is from that level. If it appears we have an attitude you are quite correct and at times it's justified. Blacks have risen above slavery, educated themselves, fought in all the major wars, participate in every industrial period, but we're painted as second rates and sadly many of us have accepted that attitude and it is shown in the way we deal each other and our attitude toward whites. This attitude is now reflected at the voting stations. I went to a special election for senator and at our voting station only 20 people voted. I hear a lot of people complaining, but no one is voting or voicing their opinion at the voting booth. For blacks this is bad because if you don't exercise your right to vote things will never change. Many blacks forget that things are the way they are because someone voted in a lot of these negative laws. And to change things we must exercise our vote. In the 50's and 60's blacks were picketing and marching for the right to vote and now 30 years later they're thinking of reasons why they shouldn't. I can look around every day and see many reasons why they should.

Many times I feel I shouldn't write about my cancer experience because I personally feel that many time no one really cares or are concern especially if you're black. I see a lot of people in the paper and on television talking about cancer and 99% of them are white; there are many of us blacks struggling with cancer and striving to lead productive lives. I talk and write about it because to me it is mental therapy that should be shared not held, and that's no matter the results.

A few months ago I was talking to a younger cousin, whom said I sound depress and I have to agree that many times I am depressed. I believe that we Blacks have bought into a negative way of thinking that is destructive to our physical and mental well-being. Some of those old teachings from slavery are still there. Things such as how we look at ourselves, how we treat each other, how we look at our future, our education, many of us feel uncomfortable about being in charge or having anything because we feel someone will try to take everything away. You can't really be positive because you will become peoples unwarranted target for abuse. The general belief is that we should take all this hate, and abuse heaped on us, as if we're playthings. This isn't something that we've taught ourselves this is something that we're encouraged to buy into by society itself.

In my attempts to be positive and rebuild my body and mind I run into a lot of depressing and negative people. I believe that when you're in the hospital many will come and see you but when you leave the hospital everything changes and the negative comes out. Now that you're home struggling to recover, everyone starts thinking about what you should do for them. I have no problem with helping people, but I ask what are you doing for yourself. You talk to people about your ideas and goals and they get bitter and say all you are concern about is yourself. And you explain that what you're doing or planning to do could benefit everyone. Basically I believe many people want a free ride. You get them a job then they want you to take them to work, get them a home they want you to clean it and cut the grass, they have kids then they want you to take care of them. One that really gets me is that when it comes time to go to work they're always sick. I become depressed YES, because here I am a cancer patient attempting to beat the odds and I find myself surrounded by negative thinkers. Even in business you find these people. They complain about how their business isn't growing and they're off doing everything but worrying about their business, they're into others business, but never their own.

Being Black you find yourself being the unwilling target of everyone's negative thoughts and ideas. If you have ideas people resist you and create barriers to stop or limit your growth, if you get beyond their barriers people will attempt to discredit you and your success. Once some type of limit success has been established and people find that they can't stop you then they want you to believe that you're responsible for them and you should have them with you. All that talk of theirs sound well, but where were they when you needed them and their support. They were negative about your ideas at the start and now they want to ride on your success, dead weight you don't need. When recovering from cancer and its evils, you find that the war is continually being fought against negative thoughts and negative thinking people. The war is being fought at home, in the hospital and on the job. To win you must believe in your goals and strive to succeed.

Do I continually think of negative things? No. I try to think positive about everything but I find that when you try to think positive and try to be constructive negative thoughts appear. You don't have to find negative idea's, negative thoughts and ideas find you. Do not dwell on ideas or inputs as negative or even evil because many things basically are not but they can go either way negative or positive. Your goal if you believe in successful completing of ideas or task is to recognize these negative and sometime hateful ideas pushing them and the barriers they create aside and press forward.

People's attitude is that now you're a recovering cancer patient you're suppose to be working on some type of social program. Assisting people I understand, but being part of some type of social agency I say no. I'm still working on my idea's and goals, and I believe anyone with dreams should continue to work on those goals. Some of my friends that I grew-up with are now dead or seriously ill not from old age, but because I believe they gave up on themselves and their ideas. They died because of illness related to drugs, alcohol, and homelessness. Many became seriously ill because they started carrying others responsibilities that can become a terrible burden becoming emotion baggage you don't need. Sometimes these people attitudes become yours, which is what they want. Their life goes on and yours go down the hill. You will need some type of foundation. My foundation is built on God and a belief in me. So as a patient of any illness you must strive to win and become healthier. Always continue to improve but watch for negative people and their ideas. You will win.

MOVING THROUGH THE TURBULENCE

Going through cancer recovery is a very emotional and turbulent time. Because in the fight to combat this disease I've found myself surrounded my negative thinkers and their attempts to have their life style ease into both my wife's life and me. Sometimes it seems no one really wants to help me and wife in achieving our goals. Bottom line is its always what we should do for everyone else personal and business wise and don't be concern about ourselves because that's not important. Everyone wants us to take on their problems and when things don't work out they say we have to help them find solution. For my wife this unnecessary pressure is taking its toll. To me it's bad enough with her being a diabetic, but because of this outside responsibility her business is failing because of neglect. Health wise, well she recently broke her foot which require surgery, her hair is thinning, she is having dental problems, she's having skin problems, recently she fell and injured her elbow and her nerves are worn thin, she has spent hundreds of dollars on gas and maintenance on her cars driving people around and no-one really shows concern. Everyone calls her at midnight and 7 o'clock in the morning asking her for solutions to their problems, never thinking of her life or business. It's fascinating how everyone wants her to drop what she is doing and do things for them. They want her to pickup their kids, drive them shopping, pickup them up at work and when there is no job they want her to help them find a job. And when you ask them about their problems they say they're too tired or they don't have transportation. When I say catch a bus everyone gets an attitude. When Frances is sick or having trouble everyone will now say they are too tired or busy.

For me my business and personal life is suffering. Health wise I question things because even though my test are coming back good I believe something maybe wrong. Physically and mentally I feel something is happening that I can't explain. Lately I've found myself awakening in the middle of the night due to sharp bone pain. I don't believe I have any broken bone but this pain I find alarming. Our rent is high and the utility bills have doubled and the bills keep coming, and everyone say that is the way it is and ask what type of deals I can give them. And I don't see any real support in sight.

I see this as an assault on our lives. I remember when my wife and I would go out to breakfast and talk about everything. Occasionally we would go out to dinner and sometimes to the movies. We would talk about all types of business. But now we do very few of these things. She said she has to take care of all these other things and I'm being selfish. Sometimes it appears that the better I get the more everyone wants to push me into a corner. My thoughts on everything can be seen in the letter I wrote my sister.

31 July 1998

Hi Joann

It's me writing and I'm fine. Yes no check. When I say I don't have any money that's what I mean. I'm tired of people talking to me like I'm some-type of money tree. I'm out here hustling my butt off trying to develop new ideas and all I get in return is a lot of crap. And that includes family. (No, not you) I'm out here paying rent, utilities, car and truck note, got a business and living in a house we can't afford and everyone is saying, I've got it made. That's bull shit I'm worse off than I was ten years ago. To live well you have to find ways to grow. To do well 10 years from now you have to look at what you're doing now, then study how things can be better.

I see a lot of money changing hands, ideas being developed and many of us Blacks being left out of the picture. Don't tell me what we have to do, because the only thing we haven't done is shot somebody. I served in the military, been to all types of schools, never been in prison and at 55 years old everyone wants to talk to me like I'm a slave or sometype of fucking idiot. The reason we blacks are in our present situation is because we believe the white masters are going to save us, as if nothing is going to change unless the whites approve. Fuck that because nothing is going to change unless we make it change. Shit, slavery ended 100 years ago and society and many Blacks are still thinking of us as slaves.

Look at Papa's farm. It was one of the largest in the area, now it's down to a measly 40 acres and everyone is arguing over that. That farm should be acting as a foundation for other things. Instead of using the tools available and making things grow, many of us believe that the only way to get something is to suck up or kiss ass.

I'm not talking foolish, take a few minutes and look at your self. Do you want to be in the same position next year or do you want things to be better. Myself, I fighting cancer, black stereotypes, family and people in general in my attempt to improve. I'm trying to kick all the bums to the curb.

Love You Always

Warren

Moving through all this turbulence I believe things will changes for the better, but first you must recognize those negative destructive things in your life and then some changes must be made by getting rid of dead weight, and recovery and growth will be smoother.

STILL WRITING

I'm still writing and trying to do things. This article is becoming a true exercise of the mind. Thinking of things to write, places to go and things to do have truly been a challenge. But I work at it.

FAMILY

Attempting to improve includes having a strong Black family. Today we see and read a lot about the deteriorating conditions of the Black family.

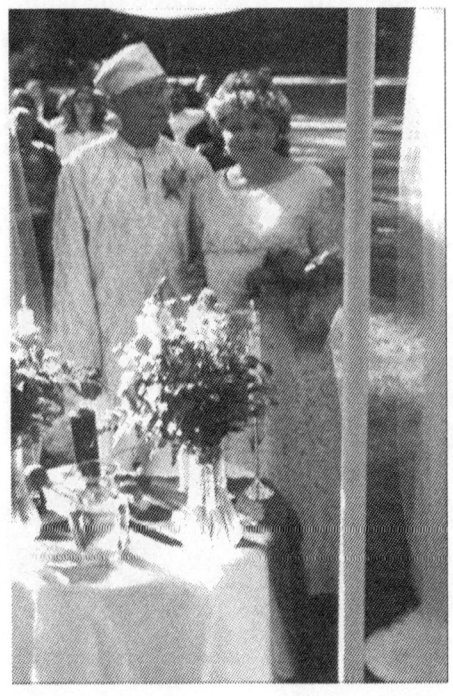

The Black family is under attack by negative image created by the media, and that includes the press. The Black community has been under attack by heavy drug. The Black male has been shown as weak and undependable and the Black female is also shown in a negative image. Black families are created everyday with strong positive head of households. Although many of us are descendent from slaves we still maintain that strong family connection with Africa and the strong community which was taught and past on my elders. Despite what many outside the Black community say, both the men and women work hard to create a strong family. While the men are working, the women are teaching. Through teaching and example they create a strong family unit. The family is

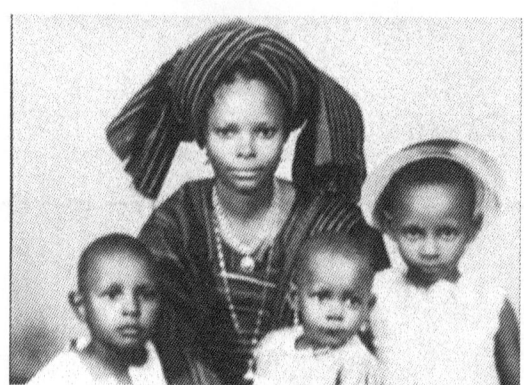

probably the strongest institute in the world. It seems as if on occasion people are trying to weaken it and if posible destroy it. Understanding how the family work some people take their family and abuse them; ever placing all their problems on them. You know the drill! Every time something goes wrong they blame the family having that selective memory they forget what they were originally taught. It seems that society pushes the blame for your problems on the family as a whole, or someone in the family and always dictating to you what your family can't do. Thus weakening the family structure. The family should be used as a positive tool for growth helping everyone to grow and move forward. It should not reflect the negative side of society, which can sometime mean death. When times are good many of us never think of family, but when things change for the worse we turn to the family for support.

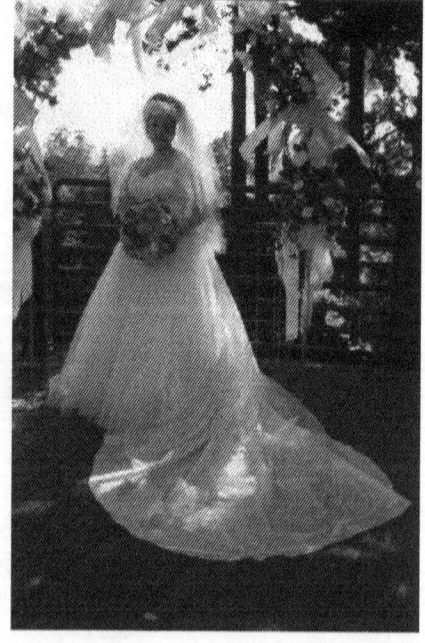

HAPPY BIRTHDAY

We just helped my brother-in-law Donald Reed celebrate his 50th birthday. The Family had a surprise party for him. And like the guest of honor he arrived late. My wife and I was surprised to see all the sisters and brothers there. Everyone brought kids and grandkids. My wife, our niece Tia and two of the sisters worked all night cooking and setting up everything. It was so many people that it was lik a family reunion. Enough money was collected that my Wife used it to buy him and his wife round trip airline tickets to his son's graduation from Brigham Young College. A man who has done almost everything, now serves as a positive role model and a motivational speaker for the family. He is still attempts to stay busy even as a kidney dialysis patient making his weekly trips to the medical center for treatment. The center has us occasionally worried because it appears that on many occasions they draw to much fluid but Don has always come through smiling. I know that with that positive attitude of his that on many instances he took me out of my slump. Yes, I have those down moments but its people like him that build me up.

All his brother-in-laws where there. His son living in the Bay Area was there. The complete party was a lot of fun with plenty of food, dancing and everyone was dancing including the little kids. One reason I think it was such a nice party was because there was no alcohol. As always someone will bring a bottle of something but most of the family are non-drinkers. Even the youngest sister and her new husband was there.

The recreation building we used was rented for us by one of the sisters. Other than a few cousins the only people that didn't show was those from Sacramento and Texas.

CHANGES THROUGH A PASSING OF TIME

As time passes many things change and this includes people and places. I think of the People, places, and events that got me this far,. These are

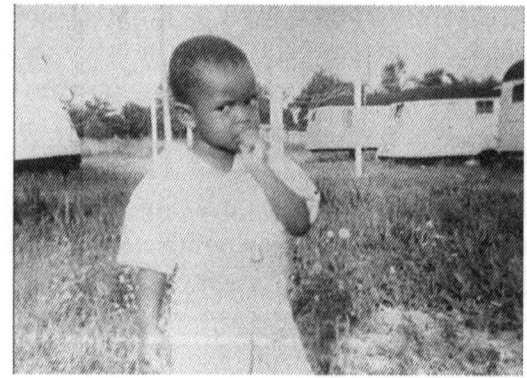

mostly events or people that mold you and spark your imagination. My first pets were a box of kittens given me by my Aunt Tippy when I was about 5 years old. I love those little animals. I remember when the doctors had removed my tonsils and my throat

was sore my father gave me a large Japanese Beetle as a pet, and he even gave me a leach so that the beetle wouldn't fly away. I was so excited I forgot that sore throat. From then on I always loved

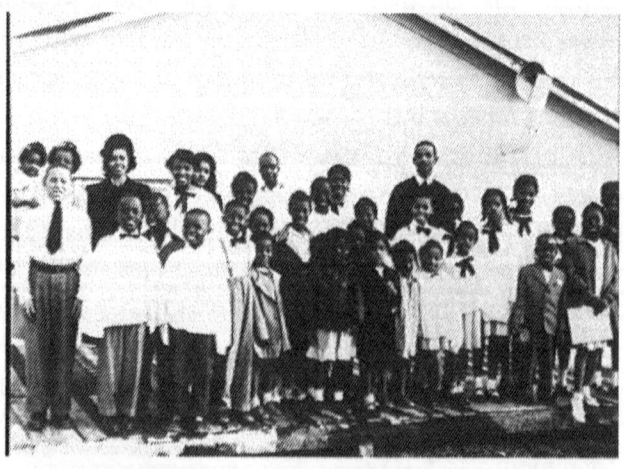

animals. I remember Reverend Stevenson building the community church from an abandon building beside a creek becoming the communities house of worship. The church was Alexander P. Shaw Methodist church now moved to higher, safer ground. In the Black community of Simms Drive housing project in Washington D.C. this became an important meeting and recreation center. I remember at eight years old attempting to cook my first egg and that was a disaster. At 9 years old building a 2 story club house behind the apartment house where my parents lived. Myself and some of the kids built it from scrap wood, after watching the grownups.

I always wanted to build and be in business. On mothers day I sold artificial flowers made by my father. After school I sold Ebony and Jet magazines and the Afro-American newspaper. On weekends I carried peoples groceries to their car or their home to earn spending money.

As a youth I remember riding the buses because an automobile was a luxury. Owning any type of Automotive machine was exciting. My uncle John had a large truck he used for hauling or moving furniture. I remember the neighborhood theater, Carver theater, seeing movies like Carman Jones, Snow White and the seven Dwarfs, and the excitement of King Kong and Creature from the Black Lagoon. And lets not forget movies like This Island Earth, and The Mystirians.

Now almost everyone has a car or truck. The price of public transportation has gone up and many fly between cities aboard Airplanes. Ships that were used to travel between countries now have holiday cruises. Military ships now have computer guided missiles instead of the antique 5 inch guns. I remember the excitement of going to the neighborhood grocery store for my mother, now many of the country or neighborhood stores have been replaced by super markets or giant shopping centers. Neighborhood theaters have been replaced with cinema complexes. And many movies now depend on special computer effects. As a youth black and white Television was a luxury now it's the computer. To relax you can now go into a local coffee shop or book store and while relaxing have a cup of coffee and a pastry.

I was always tinkering and fixing things. I would get an old bike and repair it and ride all over Washington D. C. seeing relatives and friend and going downtown to see the many sights. During the summer I would leave home early in the morning with my bike and return home late in the evening. Tinkering is something I still do especially when I'm doing repair work because I'm willing to look at things when they are broken and think of ways to repair them.

My time in high school was exciting. Although the school was a vocational school you were taught not only a skill, but you were taught business. Your normal school day started 8:30 am and on days when you had military instruction your day started at 7:30 am. As part of your training you worked on teachers homes. This was exciting because you went to neighborhood you wouldn't normally get to see. The exciting time was the High School Military Cadet Corp Competition held in Washington D.C. every year where all the city schools high school cadets competed in drill competition. Along with sports, there was also the school rifle team and the daily training at the schools rifle range. The most important day was graduation when my cousin John Jr., my friend Clifton McCray and I received our high school diploma. The school is now closed but the memories are still there.

I left home at 18 years old to join the navy. Now I was in a world of strict discipline, Traveled to Foreign countries, saw different people and listen to how they talk and watch what they do. With the passing of time you eventually have change, either in people, governments, or technology.

Going through the passing of time we are confronted with many changes. These changes are sometimes met with happiness, fear, curiosity, even hate. I've found fear is the greatest evil before me. As a cancer patient doing well, I feel people look at me more as a curiosity than a success because they were taught to believe that everything would fail. I believe

I'm doing well because over time I've taught myself to face changes with excitement and curiosity and with that attitude to always finish.

Many fear a passing of time always talking about how things were, wishing they could go back and undo the changes. To me it is fascinating watching these change. Many of these changes help and there are those that don't. Many distract you from family and community but these changes occur none-the-less. In this fight with cancer I have seen many ups and downs. Sometimes I cry because of the severity of my cancer, my friends although they stuck by me didn't believe I would survive. My doctors and nurses even though they were concern didn't think I would survive the transplant. How justified their thoughts because they knew how many times I had been admitted into emergency for cancer related problem. But I've survived and I'm glad. The thing is to not be afraid of change or severe problems but to use them as tools to help you build a better and brighter tomorrow.

DEMONS

Demon—a source or agent of evil, harm, distress, or ruin

My friend Gene and I were talking about a seminar that him and some fellow Black men attended at his home. And one of the things they talked about was confronting your demons. These demons are things in our life that hold us back. One of the men in the group who was a cancer patient felt his demon was he worked to hard, so he took a year off from work to spend with his new grandson. This was something that was important to everyone because in today's society very few people are talking to their kids or grandchildren, allowing them to be influence by outside sources such as the television. Demons, yes we all have them. The thing is to recognize them, deal with them, and deal with them but not to dwell on them. Hospital's are full of people who lost their mind continually thinking about those demons.

As a Black I find that I must fight many demons. These are negative things I been taught as I move through life. These are things that are contrary to the natural order of things. Things taught by family and friends. Subjects taught by people who want to manipulate you. For us Blacks many of our demon's go back to slavery. To me Black's are the same as everyone else with the only exception being that out of necessity we must have a strong sense of survival and competitiveness.

Where did all this start? Let's go back to the beginning of slavery here in America. Land was plentiful but there was a labor shortage there was no-one to do the back breaking work of working in the fields. Many diplomatic types needed someone to take care their personal needs or their property while they went about their daily business. There were some indenture servants, these were those who work to earn their passage to the new world, but they were in short supply.

What do you do about this shortage? How about getting slaves from Africa. The Dutch and Portuguese were very successful in this time type of trade. The suppliers being the Arab and African world. Slaves were traded like cattle. Some were for house work, some for fields, some for skilled labor and some for breeding and sexual pleasure. Slavery was a thriving business. History books sometime lie, many times they are written to please the victor. Unlike in the movies Africans weren't heathens running around in loin clothes many were educated with skill's that many in the world never possessed. When Europe was filled with barbarians, Africans had already established universities and were using the science of navigation. Picture yourself as a free person and now slavery is thrust upon you. Sure you've heard of it or even seen slaves, but now your village or town is being raided by slavers or another tribe. First the chief or elders are killed, next the sickly or wounded, and afterwards the babies. There is to be no dead weight. Now the horror begins, you are roped or lashed (chains aren't used because they are to heavy and may damage the skin during long trips)together with other captives for your long journey to the nearest shipping port you know not where, but everyone has heard stories. Over hot deserts through hostile jungle, at night you hear the sound of hungry animals. Sometimes the group would be attacked not by people, but animals, as you attempt to hide or defend yourself you see a body being dragged away clutched in the powerful jaws of an animal you know not what, and you hear the sounds of the victims helpless screams. After your long journey you arrive in a small town busy with the activities of trading. You have never seen so many people in one place, and you marvel at their skin color. You now are put in a large prison in preparation for shipping. Your cell has windows and you see all types of strange vessel floating on the water. As you look through your cell windows you see men in fine cloths arguing. You wonder, are they arguing over us their captors? During their discussion things get intense, weapons are drawn but no blood is shed. Everyone starts laughing, some type of currency changes hand, weapons are put away and everyone goes their way. You ask your jailer what is going on. His answer " Business as Usual". Now reality starts to set in your mind, you're a piece of property to be bartered and traded.

Now it's morning and you're awaken by sharp kicks and jabs. You are lead into a court yard to be inspected. Everything is being checked there is no privacy. Afterwards you are being led to a ship, destination unknown. Have you ever been to the bottom of a ship? On today's ship that's the bilge and here you find oil and water slushing about. I've worked in these area with these conditions and it's no fun. Now put yourself on those ships of wood and pitch, with little or no ventilation you are surrounded by the smell of urine and body waste, the smell of people becoming seasick, here in these dark cramp quarters there are men, women, and children. Many will die from just suffocation. Here you are tightly packed like sardines and on the decks above your tormentors are pacing up and down with guns, whips, and clubs anticipating any trouble. And if there are trouble-makers they are thrown over the side, the sea tells no tales. You're at sea for week's maybe month's because slaves aren't the only cargo, ships captains may stop in many ports transferring cargo. Even though you're confined to dark quarter you can see light through the cracks in the deck above. In rough sea's you feel the ship moving through the water, and you can hears the wave's crashing against the sides of the ship. Your stomach turns with ever pitch and roll. After all this even you believe that there is no hope.

As a supplier if your supply of slaves were low you would raid a village. The return on your money was good. Like today's merchants, once a person was captured and made a slave you took every effort to insure your product wasn't damaged. The weak, injured or wounded were destroyed. So what does that have to do with today.

Well, to control people you have to give people a feeling of there not being any hope, that you control their life, their complete existence is in your hand. You seduce people through drugs or alcohol or provide them some type jewels or currency. During times of slavery once you have control you change people through intimidation. First you use the whip, next cut off a limb, if that don't work than you kill off someone. You hang someone or drag them to pieces. No-one cares because these are slaves. Like any commodity everyone felt slaves had no rights, slaves were even taught they had no rights and their goal in life was to please others. How about that trip to America. White's had some type of habitable living quarters they may have been cramp but compared to slave quarters they were luxury. Whites talk proudly of how their ancestors came to America, Africans were never allowed this type of personal history.

Now as we approach today's time many will say that Black's are lazy, lack responsibility, poor family people and the list goes on and on. Who created this image? It certainly wasn't us Blacks. Unfortunately many of us believe these negative images and that's our problem. We're filling the jails not just because of crime but because we feel that someone must support us. Gene and I was talking about how some blacks hated for slavery to end. Why? Some slaves felt they had good masters, they didn't have to worry about their next meal, and they had clothes. During slow times in America many slaves saw whites without jobs so to them slavery wasn't bad because they had food and in the winter they had shelter so what if some were hung that's the way it was, get over it. Their only concern was hoping they had a good master. Many of the families had been apart of slavery since its start so what was the meaning of freedom. After so many years under the whip, intimidation, and just plain violent, there was no drive or ambition. The only success for being intelligent was possible death. Like animals in a circus their main concern was pleasing the overseer. When slavery ended many met freedom with no skill and no ideal of what to do. Many slipped into a new form of slavery call share croppers.

Today everyone's talking about Black's attitude, but they never look back at Blacks past, and how those attitude was developed. Have you studied Black history? Many of you will say yes, but many of you know you haven't especially whites. If you did you would know that Whites during and after slavery maintained their control over slaves or black free-man through intimidation. Starting with Washington D.C. and working across country whites destroyed Black communities and towns. In many cities there was curfews just for Blacks. Frequently Blacks were denied the right to own weapons. You were not allowed to accumulate any real wealth and if you did there was few places to spend it. Skilled Blacks were denied access to many professions that they were trained to perform. They were even denied the rights to many of their inventions we use to today. We weren't even given what many considered full Civil Rights until the sixties.

Today's society in our quest to achieve and rise above the position others created for us, Black's are now being encouraged to embrace the drug culture and its divisiveness. Today much of our thinking is based on the attitude of drug users and dealers where that enforcement of drug use and its dealings are built on a foundation taught during slavery. Whether or not we want to admit it look at the signs, they are there. All inhibitions are removed, the way we dress, talk, deal with people, and even types of crime have changed. Sure many don't use drugs, but they deal in the selling of drugs knowing the destructive power of these chemicals and the depend-ency that follows. Many ignore the use of drugs as if it's a passing thing. But to their surprise it isn't. They are shocked and surprised when a drug user mugs them or even breaks into their home. What people don't realize is that drug use is a form of slavery. Its users concern is only to please those new masters, the drug habit, and it's dealers. User's will lie, cheat, steal or even kill each other including family to please their new master.

Whether we admit it or not those demons from slavery are still with us and we must continually strive to destroy them.

ADOLESCENCE

Because of those many Demons we blacks must confront, mentally and physically we have never been allowed to mature as a social group always treated as children. Many will say that we have been given all types of opportunity. To this I say yes, but I find the opportunities are taken away or made unavailable. Skills taught become obsolete because of now non-use. The demons from slavery are still here because of many of us believe that nothing can or will happen without the white masters approval. Historically this line of thinking has been pressed upon us through all types of harassment and some of it is from the law itself. You build a town whites burn it down, you get better schools but you're given second rate books, you create a business everyone thinks of a reason to close it, You train and learn a skill and no-one wants to use them. The list is long because everyone has a reason for not working with us. During that period of slavery in this country we were placed under intense intimidation to think as a slave or servant. Because of all this training our minds, our thinking has been reduced in many instances to that of an adolescent looking up to his parents to solve all his problems. We are always talking about what others should do for us. The situation has become intense that now we question our own ability which is what many desire, because now everything stops and we never rise to the next mental level. When we complain everyone starts talking to us as if we are children, saying stop your whining. Many will say we're claiming that everyone is picking on us, and they are right. To divert things away from the issue many other social

75

groups(white females, gays and etc) are saying so what they are a minority and they are being discriminated again. I say yea get real. You're a minority because you want to set yourself apart through your actions or life style. In truth you are still part of that white main stream and the opportunity is there to blend in without any threat of reprisal. For us Blacks the opportunities are different because we are an easy group to target mainly because of skin color and facial features. No matter what happens we are easy to pick out in a crowd. Because of our skin color we are always painted as an inferior product of nature.

Looking back at Blacks past, everyone's talking about Black's attitude, but not how that attitude was developed. Because of all these demons we have never been allowed to leave adolescence and rise fully into maturity.

ETHNIC CLEANSING

Ethnic Cleansing-the elimination of an unwanted ethnic group from a society, as by genocide or forced migration.

Today America is involved in conflicts throughout the world. Attempting to stop ethnic cleansing. In Yugoslavia it's based on religion. In Africa it is based on tribal difference, and in Asia it is based on political difference. Many say we shouldn't get involved, it's their country they should be able to do what they want. I say that's a bunch of bull. What gives one group the right to kill off another just because of differences especially when everyone has sworn allegiance to that country. Many Blacks here say don't get involved, it doesn't involve us. Well, I've got news for you, those countries involved have agents here teaching that same ethnic and racial hate. We Blacks should be the 1st to speak out against ethnic cleansing, mainly because of our past history of slavery. Many African tribal groups ended up as slave do to a type of ethnic cleansing. One group wanted the other groups land, another was jealous of another's economical power, because of this a war would start and the loser would end up on the auction block. Today there is no big market for slaves, so now complete social groups are being killed. Here in America we Black's must not turn our backs because this type of hate could spread to us. There are many here who hate us and if they had the power would start killing us or put us back in slavery. We can't sit like idols thinking some-one else or God is going to take care of things, there are something's we must do ourselves. If you don't than you must believe you are a slave and your master will take care of everything. Your training as a slave was very good and it's reflected in your attitude. Well, I have news for you if you don't get involve you might find yourself back with a master and he might be worse than the last. Evil is always at work and we must confront it and say enough is enough. Why? Because those Demons from slavery still exist and they are popping up everywhere.

A Slave

I went to sleep last night a free man, and awaken this morning a slave.

What a statement to make but indeed it is a true statement. Having cancer gives me a chance to think to read and ask questions. Basically it gives me a chance to think and collect my thoughts and put everything in order. Slavery has been dead for more than a hundred years and that's along time, but for the slavery issue it isn't. As a contractor I had one regular customer whose grandfather fought for the confederacy during the civil war and it was a pleasant experience working with him and his family. Slavery is only three generations away which isn't very far. And for us Blacks that's terrible or I should say horrifying. Why? Because everything being taught out there in the real world when dealing with black/white issues is based on information collected during, before or directly after slavery and the information collected, written, and circulated was controlled by whites. All information circulated is based on our being inferior and when we differ our society go into denial and that's black and white. Yes, many blacks go into denial because they don't want to upset the status quo. This I don't understand because these same people are complaining about how Blacks are being treated. Well, actually I do because these same people are looking for power and clot and they feel that if they can show whites that they can control or maneuver black people than whites will give them some type of position of power. For us Blacks that's scary because once in power instead of treating us as equals, to the rest of the world they treat us as inferiors.

Sometimes it's nice being an observer, because I can see all the negative teachings being passed on to the next generation. Many of us are passing on information that is chaotic and none productive. Look at the way we dress, the way we talk, the way we carry ourselves. And many of us feel comfortable with whites in charge. I don't have a problem with whites or any other social group in charge, but many of us put them up on that pedestal for all the wrong reasons. To many blacks they feel that nothing will go right unless a white is in charge. They forget that no Blacks destroyed a nation with nuclear weapons, created biological weapons or killed off millions of people the way the Germans did during the Second World War. Sure Blacks and black nations have problems but their biggest problem is mimicking the whites. It's almost as if they believe even though they're free they still must please their imaginary white master. So de facto slavery is still here.

As I look at cancer, I wonder why the treatment of it wasn't encouraged more in the past in the black community. The Bone Marrow Program has been going on for more than 20 years and the medical fields are just starting to really push for donors in the Black community. What happened with the medical field, did they feel that the whites were the only one's worth saving. How many Blacks died of A.I.D's before someone started working on a treatment. That slavery thinking is still here and for everything to improve across the board for everyone we will have to make a change.

A Black Mans Dilemma

Given Equal Rights under the law, but denied equal access to the law
That's the way it is, Get over it
Given Equal Opportunity without the equal
That's the way it is, Get over it
Allowed to live anywhere, but still must remain in the shadows
That's the way it is, Get over it
Work anywhere but always seen as labor
That's the way it is, Get over it
Allowed to request a bank business loan, but left at the Tellers window
That's the way it is, Get over it
Open a business but criticized for wanting to be better
That's the way it is, Get over it
Allowed in the office, but always left by the water fountain
That's the way it is, Get over it
Always told how good you are, but never allowed to be number one
I know, THAT'S THE WAY IT IS, GET OVER IT
Yes I'll get over it, but will you like the change

NIGGAR

American Definition: Niggar-Referring to a Black person as less than or having little worth. Persons considered as second class or possessing a lower intelligence.

I noticed some young black kids seven and eight years old calling each other and referring to some other kids as niggars. Why are we (Blacks) teaching our kids to hate themselves or allow others to create an atmosphere of doubt, where youth question their self worth as a person and an ethnic group? I remember as a youngster that if you called someone niggar it was an insult which resulted in a fight. It's still spoken as an insult but it's become common place especially in the black community. Some of the pride in being black has been lost because instead of working to build ourselves up many of us are striving to prove to others and ourselves that we are the lowly figures people believe us to be. How can you get respect if you're not demanding respect from yourself.

Niggar or Nigger is a title that was tagged to Slaves and freed Blacks during the time of Slavery. It is easier to call you niggar than recognize your ethnic history. The name was really pressed on us after slavery to show you who is in charge. Now who is in charge of your life? Slavery has been dead over a hundred years. Look at yourself, give yourself a mental work over. Do you give the appearance of being embarrass about who you are, You know the dropped head, drooping shoulders. Does your clothes appear to be falling off you? Sure it's the style, but whose style? Do you take drugs and alcohol? Why? Is this your way of feeling accepted even if it means getting so drunk or high that you pass out in front of kids awakening with a foul body smell. Are you one of those people that feel so poor of yourself that to lift yourself up you have to use a lot of profanity to bring everyone down to your level. Many Blacks notice how people (Black and White) when engaged in conversation with us speak or treat us as if we're children. And that attitude is reflected everyday in how we as a people view ourselves. How many times have you seen grown men and women acting and dressing as if they're kids, many want us to even take on their responsibilities, and when we don't they have a temper tantrum.

Remember many of us Blacks although descendent of slaves, came from a group of proud people. They didn't volunteer to come here, they were forced. Slaves were obtained through village raids or tribal warfare(that activity continue today but since there is no slave market they kill off each other). No-one asked for tickets to America. So, remember no niggars were brought to this country just Africans.

BLACK MAN'S TEARS

Oh, ungrateful nation
How you forget about
that other nation in America,
Oh yes, Black America
Over three hundred years ago
we were snatched from our home.
Next we were forced into servitude,
Bringing nothing, we were denied any history,
any family, any education and no social status except that of slave or
servant.
Yes, there were free blacks but the same basic rules and laws applied,
we were still considered less than.
We were hanged, murdered and raped. Sometimes for nothing less than
looking wrong at someone. If we showed a gleam in our eyes that was
enough to be whipped.
Oh, the tears.

We were always taught to believe that our life, our destiny was
controlled by others. How foolish can one get?
We were trained and taught by everyone including the Black community
to believe that it
is alright for someone to treat you this way, as if you are some type of pet.
After slavery our towns and communities are destroyed sometimes for
no other reason

than to set an example for others.

Many of our hero's are gone. Destroyed in many ways. Some by hanging many by assassination. Even today many are lost through broken spirit. The weight of striving and the resistance that ensues becoming too great.

Oh, the tears

Now free we're suppose to have equal rights.
We have been part of the development of America
We have fought in every war,
but things have not changed.
We are still taught and teaching that someone else controls our destiny,
That it is fine to be treated as we are.
After over a hundred years of freedom, and struggle, like children we still must explain
why we want or should have things.
No matter our success our ability is still questioned by everyone including ourselves.
We complain about prison, but we teach our kids that it's alright to go to jail.
We say we have pride but we are still looking down at ourselves.
Oh, the tears, have nothing changed.
These aren't tears of hate, bitterness, or even malice,
these are tears of concern.
Many ask when will this hatred end?
The answer is never if you refuse to take hold of your future.
The time now is to take hold of power and make the changes,
not being concerned about others, because in the political arena as in life people will criticize no matter what you do.
In taking charge
and making those positive changes then will the Black Man's Tears stop.

THE INTERVIEW

Warren G.H Fisher Jr

My name is Clarence Hinkle and this is my interview with Mr. Oswald King the Blackman considered the financial backer for many of the

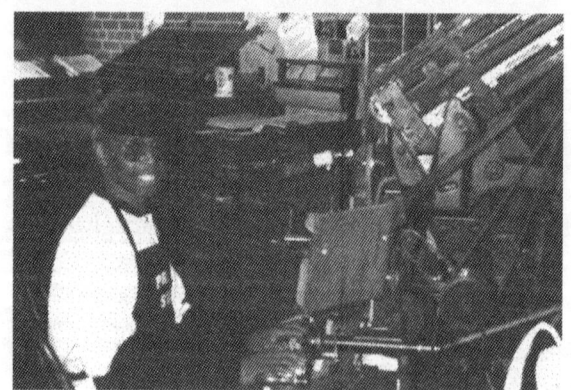

Black organizations in America.

Good morning Mr. King

Good Morning

I see through my list that you supposedly back many Black organizations, some considered violent. May I ask Why?

I do finance many Black organizations, but none are violent. The only people that view them as violent are some Blacks, but mostly whites, because here are blacks that are not part of that group that is considered normal. Look around my friend at the Black society. I ask you this question how far have we come from slavery? Looking at the era since the civil rights movements many times it appears we are moving backwards.

Mr. King, how or should I say why did you get involve in civil rights?

Well, it goes back to my grandparents. My grandfather was killed by another family member and that took a mental toll on my grandmother.

The family later admitted her in a home. Plus other more important reasons. Now what does that have to do with civil rights? As a Black you're taught to hate self and family. So if you have a problem it is fine to kill another Black or Family, but kill a white, man you're in real trouble. I've also seen or read of how Blacks have been beaten or killed for being too intelligent and this must end.

Mr. King, What is your education Level?

Well, I have a degree in engineering, I speak 10 languages, and I've lived in 4 countries.

Mr. King with all this travel how did you start your many businesses? It appears your interest is everywhere.

Well, after serving in the Military, and finishing college I did a lot of traveling. After returning to America I started investing in any and everything and it paid off. My businesses which still are in operation today I had to have whites front for me, but now the businesses are all run by family.

Mr. King, from the stories I've heard it seems that you have been around forever I know everything can't be true. Because you look 60 years old.

Well, everything you have heard is true. Before I start, I suggest you have a cup of coffee or a drink.

No thank you

I suggest you do, I'll go and have my daughter prepare something, excuse me.

May I look around, these pictures and artwork look so old are they real?

Yes

I rose from my chair and walked about this great room. The room is about the size of most Black peoples homes. How can a Black man have such a large home and live such a quiet life. I saw original art work from every point on the globe and the furniture, when you sat in a chair you felt as if it was embracing you. Driving up to his house that was a tour in it self. The house was a mile from the street, with tall hedges protecting the view. I thought I was in England visiting some dignitary. When I rang the doorbell this big guy greeting me, saying Mister King was expecting me and Miss Johnson would take me to him. Miss Johnson was the most beautiful Black woman I had ever seen and with such perfect English. I wonder what country was she native. When I met Mr. King I didn't know what to expect. Here was a man 6' tall in good physical condition with lightly gray hair his skin the color of black coffee. And now I'm interviewing him.

Well, now he is back with Miss Johnson and she is serving us coffee and cake. As she walks past I catch the fragrance of her perfume, wow, it makes your mind wander.

Mr. Hinkle lets get back to our interview. Miss Johnson is my Daughter by my third wife.

Oh! Why does he call her Miss Johnson?

Now you wonder how old I am. Well I'm well over a hundred. I was born in the south during slavery and my family escaped to the north. I fought in the Civil War. During that time I was assigned to a medical field hospital to carry bodies. There Doctor King saw me and asked me if I wanted to work with him. This to me was exciting. Here I was until the end of the war. After the war I had many jobs before the doctor again found me. He told me of some experiments he was doing and he needed me to help him with his work and to be part of his experiments. Hey, this sounded great, meals, a place to sleep, and travel. What I didn't realize was that he was working on some type of medical life enhancer. The doctors research required us to do some traveling and we finally found ourselves in Africa. There was this tribe that seem to live forever, and after years of searching we found them. What everyone said about these people was true. After numerous meetings they finally agreed to teach us everything, but first I had to be become a member of the tribe, the doctor because he was white was made some type of priest. Does that tribe exist today, yes. All my wives are from that tribe and so is everyone that works in my home. Now back to the story. Once told everything the doctor needed a test subject and that was me. The doctor had taught me everything about the medical field, so there was no problem working with him. How did you know anything was working? Your skin and facial features start changing, you become more alert, and the list goes on. The doctors didn't take it because he was to old. Shortly after returning to the states the good doctor died. But, before his death he made some type of arrangements so that the house and all his finances would go to me. So here over eighty years later you are talking to me.

Why are you telling me everything?

That's simple, the tribal council told me 40 years ago of your arrival.

So why are you supporting these Black activities or groups?

The council wants me to support Black growth, because something evil is out there and it is still attempting to keep Blacks in bondage. You see it everywhere. There is doubt, confusion, self hate, the disruption of families, lose of confidence, and low self-esteem. All these things are enhanced by drugs, violence and supported by the media.

Have you been satisfied by the results?

The answer is yes, but there has been times when we have put money on the wrong horse, as many will say.

This is hard to believe, here I am talking to a man well over a hundred, but he looks and acts 60 years old.

Maybe this will help. Miss Johnson give Mister Hinkle his folder.

My folder?

Yes your folder

As I read the material in the folder my heart started racing, here was my family history going back over a hundred year.

So I asked who has been keeping this information?

The tribal council. They keep tract of all its lost children.

So the interview ends.

Now I'm back at my office working on another story. In comes my secretary Miss Johnson with another assignment. Since the interview I get regular assignments and pay checks from persons unknown and Miss Johnson is always there as my keeper.

THE TICKETS

Warren G. H. Fisher, Jr.

What a morning

I look outside my bedroom window and all I see is snow.

My room is chilly, I'll have to check my furnace in the basement, because lately the pilot has been going out. I hear Miss Johnson downstairs. Miss Johnson is neither mistress or housekeeper, but she keeps my life in order. Since my interview with her father five years ago she has always been with me. Slender almost six feet tall she has acted as my bodyguard, cook, and secretary. The only thing she doesn't do is drive. I think that's to give me something to do.

Miss Johnson could you fix me some coffee?

Yes, would you like some breakfast

yes, but don't make the toast so dark

I'll just sit here and read the paper. Let me turn on the radio

Our ball team just won another game, more news about the president, and new intercity problems.

Now I'm in the bathroom shaving my chin. This is really something almost forty five and still don't have to shave the side of my face. This is a daily routine splashing cold water on my face and some after shave lotion.

Now I'll leave to go to the office

In route to the Office I stopped and get some donuts and a thermos of coffee. I love Krispy Kreame donuts.

Now in the office I check the mail. There are the usual, bills and checks for articles written. Here is something unusual 2 tickets for two to a town in the mid-west.

Looking at all my reference books and maps I could find nothing about this town. I ask Miss Johnson if she had any information she said no.

Well, I'll just have to wait and see.

Now 2 weeks later Miss Johnson and I are at this small modern airport. It's a regular airport with the regular activity of planes coming and going but with one notable difference, there are no whites here.

I spoke to Miss Johnson about everything and she only smiled. I believe she knows something about this town.

A car pulls up, a window goes down, and a voice says Mr. Hinkle and Miss Johnson

Yes

Get in please and I'll put your baggage in the trunk

After putting our bags in the car, the man got in and started driving.

Good morning, my name is Russell and I want to welcome you. I'll be your driver during your stay.

Russell, this is an unusual town, how long has it been here?

The town is about one hundred and fifty years old, but that will be explain to you later. I must first take you to the hotel.

Riding through town I got to see a blend of the old and new. There was old houses beside five story buildings and nothing seem out of place.

Arriving at the hotel, it was a huge 5 story piece of artwork, the plaque at the door said it was built in 1919. The structure looked as if it had come Europe. Inside everything looked as if it came from the Mediterranean or Africa.

Once Miss Johnson and I checked in we went down to the dining room and had dinner. Our table was by the window where we had a view of the people and activity on the street. For a town in the middle of nowhere there was a lot of activity. There was a regular transit system and the latest cars and trucks. As in many cities there was the sight of children riding their bikes on sidewalks. After dinner I went to my room and prepared for the days ahead and got some missed sleep.

Two days later here I am talking to the town mayor. To me this complete trip has been exciting. I visited stores, restaurants, I was even invited into homes for dinner or coffee. Everything felt like coming home. Neat homes, well kept lawns, horse and wagons, electric street cars, farm machinery, and factories everything for a prosperous town.

I'm now talking to the mayor and Miss Johnson is taking notes.

Mr. Mayor, I was given an assignment to come and speak with you. May I ask why?

You can relax Mr. Hinkle this is more for your information. The tribal council wanted you to have this information because it is needed for your mental growth.

The tribal council is part of this town?

Yes, this town is part of one Tribe and there are many towns like this throughout America. Though small we are many. Everyone living here is from that tribe. The tribe goes back over 3,000 years. We have followed and recorded man's activities thru out history.

How many people know of you, because I can't find this town on the map?

Quite a few. There are the Amish, the Quakers, many of the Native American tribes, many nations in Asia and those at home in Africa.

Whew, I had no idea. How do you keep track of everyone and everything?

The Mayor smiled and pointed to the wall and many images appeared from scenes around the world. Images seem to just appear as if the wall was alive. You felt as if you were in whatever image you viewed. An image spoke, welcome Mr. Hinkle from our deep sea habitat we hope you enjoy your visit to our modest community. The habitat is presently located in the deepest part of the Pacific ocean.

Mr. Hinkle, I see you are startled. Our technology is well in advance of today's science and our laws require us to stay that way. Much of our technology never leaves our community, we've found over history many have used our technology for a destructive nature and that was not our original intention. But, there have been moments in American history where we had to participate. The first heart surgery was done by one of our people.

I hope you and Miss Johnson enjoyed the tour of the town?

Yes I did, but I believe Miss Johnson knows more about this town

Yes she does! You know she likes you, no rush but you should marry her. Now Mr. Hinkle about this town.

Here we have a fully functioning town. We address it as our city. We are the Black Wall Street. Nothing happens in America without our knowledge. Like any city we must have a financial base. Our income come from many sources, but we cannot become involved in anything illegal or what we consider immoral. We cannot participate in anything that will bring our brother down.

Mr. Mayor, I see many factories and farms. Who owns these properties and business?

We own everything here, now much of our work is subcontracted to us by other businesses, but, the businesses here are owned by us.

Now I know it's not quiet like this all the time.

Oh! We had our moments. As with many societies, families will leave, but after a time they return.

We have social problems just like everyone, but we have our social rules to govern us.

Mr. Mayor, what about education?

Well, our education is some of the best in the world. Our youth complete school at the 10th grade and after finishing school many are sent outside of the country for further education. You will find most of the people here speak at least 4 languages, many speak 10 or more.

What about outsiders?

Very few pass through our town. We had a problem in 1919 when some whites finding out how well we were doing raided and totally destroyed our town, killing at least 300 of our people. We rebuilt our town with help from our tribal nations. The whites who attempted to destroy our town and dreams we no longer fear. Neither them or their town exist.(smile)

It is really nice to see a true Black community and not a ghetto

Mr. Hinkle, a ghetto you won't find here. The Black Ghettos, these are area's set aside for rental to Black tenant's. Now, many talk of these area's we speak of as the hood, but they are nothing more than concentration camps or reservations, where your life style is controlled by absentee landlords, and you are encouraged not to vote or complain for fear of reprisal such as eviction or raised rent. Fear is used as a major distraction to justify things such as criminal activity, and jail is seen by many as a rite-of-passage. Blacks wanted integration, but when it came instead of actively competing against white businesses they abandon their own. Many times they become angry with whites, and then they riot and burn down their own homes. What is that all about? To many they appear foolish, because now even though they may rent their homes, now with their homes destroyed they truly have nothing, but their landlord can still return to the warmth and security of his home. Shouldn't it be the reverse? Whites have Blacks train quite well, we compromise even in our anger. With this compromise our position still remains the same and like children we're soothe with a few coins. A community is where everyone share a common interest including the ownership of property, politic's and growth. Here pride is reflected in appearance of self, your home, and neighborhood. Here just because you are poor doesn't mean you have to look and act that way because you still believe there is light at the end of the tunnel. There is nothing illegal about being poor, but it is wrong to justify your continuing to be poor. Momentarily you can be poor due of the changes of time, but even that can be corrected.

Here we have a community.

After a 2 hour discussion about everything, the latest social events, politics, and the economy our interview ended. Since we still had a few more days before leaving he suggested we see the sights.

Russell our driver was there to drive us back to the hotel. On our way back I saw a sign saying museum

Russell, that museum sure looks interesting could you drop us off.

Sure. What time do you want me to pick you up.

Don't bother we will walk balk to our hotel.

After watching our limousine leave we walked into the museum.

Upon entering a well dress young man gave Miss Johnson and I a tour guide booklet showing us where everything was located. The booklet was unusual, it felt warm to the touch and it started speaking as you began walking. Who ever heard of a talking piece of paper. What strange world have we entered.

The Book answered, the world of family, of truth

Startled I dropped the book and Miss Johnson started laughing

Mr. Hinkle pick me up, this floor is cold, your official indoctrination has now started.

The nation started over 3,000 years ago in central Africa. Long before all the great powers, long before Europe and China. We were flying and sailing ships. Animal you call wild we domesticated. We worked with everyone, The Inca's with their great temples, Egypt with its great pyramids, China with the great wall, and the English with the Stone-henge. We traded around the world. Seeing the devastating affect our technology was having on the world we in time became isolationist. Now we only intervene when a threat to social order appears. Now look around and enjoy.

Miss Johnson and I spent what seemed like hours viewing everything. We asked the book a million question. We saw simple tools and the most advanced. There was computers never seen in any store or any government project. There was ships and space craft that actually worked.

I asked the Book where have these spacecraft been?

His reply, name a planet. The nation has been doing space exploration for over a century.

Our tour ended, we walked back to our hotel.

While walking I looked up at the stars and I asked Miss Johnson if those spacecraft we saw were real?

She said yes. A craft similar to the one in the museum she piloted to Pluto twenty years ago.

Well, I better quit while I'm ahead.

I wonder how it would be to take Miss Johnson out for dinner and dance, no work. Well it was just a thought.

Back at the hotel I went to my room to organize my notes and prepare for tomorrow.

Hum, this is really a nice morning. The sun ease thru the window, you can view the birds and on the street activity is everywhere.

An invitation was left at my room door inviting Miss Johnson and I to the towns festival and parade which starts at 11:00. Before going anywhere I'm going to have breakfast.

I met Miss Johnson in the dining room. For breakfast we ordered the house special. And it was a special. Breakfast starteding with soup, a carafe of juice and a pot of coffee. Next there was food brought on plates as big as platters and after trying to eat everything, they ask if we wanted dessert. I don't think so. It was a pleasant way to start the morning.

A crowd was congregating in the street, banners were flying everywhere, and music was coming from the orchestra in the town square. As the parade started, it like many parades started with the school bands, and drum majors. After that everything changed, there were dancers from all over the globe in their native dress, next there was cowboys and cowgirls driving cattle, next there was lion and tigers not in cages but walking freely and no one was afraid. Next some of the exhibits from the museum were also in the parade, and more unusual sights were always appearing. I ask one of the viewers is this an annual parade?

Yes, this is just one of many.

So, there we were spending our day watching the parade, eating all types of food and participating in the many events. In all the excitement Miss Johnson pulled me close and smile.

When we return to the hotel Miss Johnson kiss me on the cheek, and smiling said thank you for a pleasant evening.

Smiling as I went to my room I thought to myself, I will sleep good tonight.

It is now morning. Russell drove us to the airport in the limo. Now on the plane, Miss Johnson's hand resting on mines, I think how sad, because now I must become an ordinary person. But I smile because Miss Johnson and I will be back next year.

THE MYSTERY AIRCRAFT

Warren G. H. Fisher, Jr.

Ring, Ring, Ring

Who in the world is ringing my door bell this early in the morning. It's seven o'clock and I haven't even had my morning cup of coffee or my ritual bath. Miss Johnson won't answer the door, because she is doing her morning exercises; we have been working together for seven years and nothing interferes with that morning ritual.

Yes, Miss Johnson and I are still together.

Let me see whose ringing my door bell.

Good morning Doc. What are you doing here so early?

Doc is an amazing person. A quiet soft spoken man, he is a member of the tribal counsel. Because he is not one of the world's best dressed men, you would never believe he was performing open heart surgery at the age of 19 years old. Now he is here at my door.

Good morning Clarence, it's really nice out today. You should attempt to get up earlier. Where is Miss Johnson? I know, she is doing her morning exercises. Marvelous woman.

Ok Doc, What's going on?

Clarence, the council wants you and Miss Johnson to take a trip in the Pacific.

Where?

To one of our deep sea habitats.

Apparently they have been doing some scientific development and I imagine they want you to see their latest project. Here are two tickets, You and Miss Johnson will be flown to Oakland, California where you will meet our deep sea vessel.

I must leave now, I have a lot of errands today.

Have a good day Doc.

After Doc left I call to Miss Johnson. Miss Johnson, Doc left us with some airline tickets for tomorrow, apparently we have a ship to catch.

Arriving in Oakland was uneventful. We had to pick up or disembark passengers at a couple of airports en route. I slept most of the trip. My seat was by the wing; which is something I hate because I can always sense when the engines are changing speed. A car was waiting at the Airport when we arrived. It immediately took us to the ship.

Arriving at the pier, I guess I was expecting a weather battered old hulk, something out of those movies. Instead I found a sleet modern vessel about 200' long, with some type of landing area at the rear or the stern. I wonder what lands there?

This is an unusual ship named after a great African king, King Kinta. The hull was smooth, with no visible smoke stack or even radar. After coming aboard and being shown our berthing, we were given a tour. This ship was the first in its class. Although a machine it was treated as a living being that interacts with people. The ships computers name was Asoaws. The ship has a crew of 50 and it can repair and defend itself. It has a top speed of 60 plus knots. It can submerge to the deepest point in any ocean. At that moment I was startle by a shaking of the ship. Seeing the look on my face Miss Johnson told me that the ship was now getting underway.

Miss Johnson suggested that we should go on the ship's bridge and watch everything

It was amazing, how our ride was so smooth even in open rough sea. I later learned that the ship incorporated stabilizing fins which automatically adjusted to sea conditions.

Once underway Miss Johnson and I went up on the main deck and sat in lounge chairs, soaking in the sun catching the breeze as the ship moved through the water.

Eight days out we received an emergency message, an airplane was down and we're the nearest vessel

Over the intercom system word was passed to clear the decks and prepare to dive.

This was fascinating because the hull of the ship expanded and completely enveloped the ship.

Miss Johnson and I went to the bridge to see what was going on. There, we were directed to a communication and information center. Sensors were set at maximum range of 300 miles, our speed was 55 plus knots. Captain Katiro, the ships commanding officer informed us that a plane had crash and we were to check for survivors. We would be in the area in three hours. The ships computer had already launched probes that would check the area for the wreckage or any survivors and the planes black box.

Riding a ship of this type was unusual. Unlike submarines in the movies that are completely sealed with no view of the sea, here we were completely submerged and I could view the ocean around us. Cruising at very deep depths I was now able to observe sea life that was only talked about.

Miss Johnson pulled my arm

Yes?

We are entering the crash site, and the probes are checking for survivors.

The woman checking the sensors said survivors were found, about 30.

Although submerged the ship launched recovery craft which went to the surface and began picking up survivors.

We're now looking for the black box.

Looking at the planes wreckage with cameras and probe, the Captain directed the executive officer Commander Obongo, Miss Johnson, and my attention to an unusual hole in fuselage. There appeared to have been an explosion or impact on that plane. He directed the ship to move over the wreckage and recover the damage area and bring it aboard. Something unusual happened here, was it sabotage?

The recovery craft was bringing the last of the survivors aboard and the bodies of the casualties, when the ship announced unidentified ships were approaching.

The approaching ships refuse to identify themselves, these were combat ships that flew no identifiable flag.

We again asked that they identify themselves with no reply.

The officer in communication central, Lieutenant Na Lubwanna announced that a message was coming from one of the unidentified vessels, demanding that we turn over all the survivors and wreckage.

The Captain said I don't think so. What country are they?

There was no response.

Mr. Hinkle, I want you and Miss Johnson to check all information traffic on this aircraft.

Miss Johnson and I went to the Auxiliary Communication room and started checking the computers world wide. To our surprise we found that this was a government mission en route to Asia for an important conference. What was more shocking, is that the news media was already stating that the plane was lost and there were no survivors. Where were they getting their information?

At that moment the ship shook. What is going on? We rushed up to the bridge, and filled the Captain in on our information.

The Captain smiled and then directed the ship to go down to 2000 feet.

The ships had launched torpedoes, I guess to encourage us to surface. But our ship had launched some type of counter measures, using the probes that were already launched.

I asked the Captain if something could be done about the ships above?

Yes, but I don't want to start an international incident. There is something going on here and I would like to find out what.

He then directed Miss Johnson and I to go below and question some of the survivors. Because the answer is there and answers we need now.

We check the passengers, using the passenger list that came over the communication system and found the Chairman of the mission missing. We went with the ships doctor to the temporary morgue and found the chairman's body. Examining his body we found a gun shot wound.

On the way down the ladder to the dinner area where the survivors were located we heard a loud noise like a gun shot and scuffle. When we entered the dining area the crew and passengers had overpowered two people and were now securing them with handcuffs.

The surviving passengers and the plane's crew members said these people did not belong to them. How they got on the plane no one knows but, they do know that the problems with the plane started when these people went to the after section of the plane. And when the plane crashed, they had that confident attitude that everything was alright. We asked about the trade mission and was told it was important because when the trade agreements were signed it would bring stability to many of the African nations. This was important because many of these nations had been at war with each other for fifteen to twenty years. Now it appeared someone wanted to stop the signing of those papers. We took the two prisoners ID papers and went to the auxiliary computer room to verify their identity. There we found these identification papers were false, that the two were hired assassins wanted world wide for a long list of crimes. One man was an explosion expert from Asia and the other a hired gun from Europe. We notified the crew below and they placed the prisoners in the ships brig.

Miss Johnson and I returned to the Bridge and notified the Captain of the situation. About that time the ship was hit by three shock waves from detonated torpedoes.

The Captain turned to the computer Asoaws and told it to bring in all probes and make full speed for the Philippines and notify our people there of the situation. And put those nuisance ships out of action. As the ship was building speed it launched some type of weapons. The weapons were neither torpedo or missile, but they were fast. They hit those ships with a loud explosion.

The Captain turned to me smiling, don't worry they aren't sunk just stopped. We will stay submerged most of the trip just in case there are some more antagonistic crafts in the area. Our top speed is well in excess of 65 knots, for now is a need for haste.

We remained submerged for several days. About two hours before arriving in port our ship finally surfaced. Upon surfacing we were immediately met by a sister ship, King Matesa. The difference was that the ship was rigged for combat, this was strictly a combat vessel. It's mission was to insure the prisoners were delivered without any incidents.

We arrived in port early in the morning amid a crowd of photographers, reporters, television cameras, and ambulances. Also on the pier was the military police who immediately took the prisoners in custody and the plane wreckage was removed by aviation inspectors. While the captain and the local authority took care of paper work and the political protocol, Miss Johnson and I went into town and did some quick shopping.

Hours later we are back aboard ship and the ship is now underway. Now walking on the main deck en route to the main dining area, we hear laughter, and music. As we enter the dining room we see a banquet set at the main table, Women entered not in uniforms but, in native dress, with trays of food. At each table there were colorful centerpieces and floral arrangements. This was really something to see.

The menu consisted of:

Lamb Dices, Tartar Steak, Fresh Fish in Honey Sauce, Roasted Shredded Beef, Oysters Mombasa

Monrovian Collards and Cabbage, Rice and Greens

Vegetable Stew

Spicy Salad, Chopped Egg Salad

Puree of lamb Khartoum(soup) and Coconut Bean Soup.

For dessert there was Peanut Ice Cream, Fresh Pineapple with Honey, Fruit Squash, Creme Caramela and Fruits of Africa Pie.

And let us not forget the beverages! There was Cinnamon Tea, Angolan Coffee, Zambezian Tea, and Kilimanjaro Coffee.

The menu was outstanding.

After the meal there was entertainment. As the crew laughed and sang in the Dining area, Miss Johnson and I went up to the main deck. and while listening to the music coming from below Miss Johnson and I pleasantly dance the night away as the ship sails into the sunset toward our original destination.

VACATIONING IN GREECE

Warren G. H. Fisher, Jr.

It's me, Clarence Hinkle. I've finally got some time off and now here I am sitting in my lounge chair enjoying the sun on one of Greece beautiful white beaches. I've traveled up and down the Peloponnese. I've spent time in Sparta, the ancient city of Mystras, the caves of Duros. There were villages on the side of mountains, in these modern times they appeared as something time forgot. The food here is delicious. There was the Greek salad with Olive oil, Kalamata olives, feta cheese. Cheese pies (tyropita), roasted lamb, spinach pie(spinakopita), souvlaki, baked chicken. I had pastries such as kourabedes, and baklava. What a pleasant vacation.

Miss Johnson is still in the states holding down the office. So now here I am listening to Greek music, with my eyes closed enjoying the warm breeze coming off the Mediterranean. Miss Johnson and I have been working together for many years. Many times we appear as one. As a writer I have been everywhere in the world. I've help recover ancient tribal artifacts in China. In Africa, Miss Johnson and I evaded angry tribesman as we rescued some of our surviving tribesman and their families from their destroyed village. Although our tribe is strong many times our small outpost do come under attack from other tribes. Then there was the time during an at sea rescue where I was almost wash over board. What an experience, hearing giant waves hit the side of the ship and looking up helplessly seeing a wave picked me up and carried me from one side of the ship to the other. Hey, these are all experiences you never forget. Hiding in manmade tunnels, running through tall grass, and rocky creeks to evade possible capture.

How far I've come from being a kid in the projects. How times have changed especially in the Black projects. Many of us Black kids were reaching out mentally, but no-one was there. I remember at 13 years old attempting to build a nuclear reactor from drawings in books. Building a crystal radio at 11 years old that operated without batteries. Using my chemistry laboratory in my bedroom to test everyone for diabetes. Creating my own soft drink. There was Clifton and his brother Allen with their larger chemistry and biology laboratory in their bedroom. They experimented with animals. Clifton even stuffed some of his trophies. You never forgot Allen, not because of the lab, but because he liked mayonnaise and jelly sandwiches. We like kids everywhere liked playing sports and singing in the church choir. Clifton broke his leg a couple of times playing football. Many of us rode bicycles as a group, worked at the golf course, or worked on fish boats. In high school there was the class competition in spelling with students like Barbara Jordan. Barbara and I would always be the only students left, and our English teacher Mrs. Snowden would always declare a draw. In national automobile design contest there were students like Benjamin Brady who design futuristic cars, and in the schools shop class there was teachers like Mr. Hull teaching us to design model boats that actually worked..

Since then I've learn 4 languages, I've been in countries where the governments have been overthrown not once, but several time. I seen governments take people from their homes just because they looked or act guilty.

Has my life been boring? No it hasn't, it has been a growing experience. As a Black it has helped me step away from what people consider the norm for the Black community. Now here I am enjoying the sunny beaches of Greece. Miss Johnson and the council will find other assignments for me. Until then I 'll enjoy myself. So, have a good day.

BLACK COWBOYS

I know everyone remembers the white cowboys like John Wayne, Gene Autry, Roy Rogers, Red Ryder and a host of others that we saw on the big screen and television. Movies and books show Blacks as working the fields

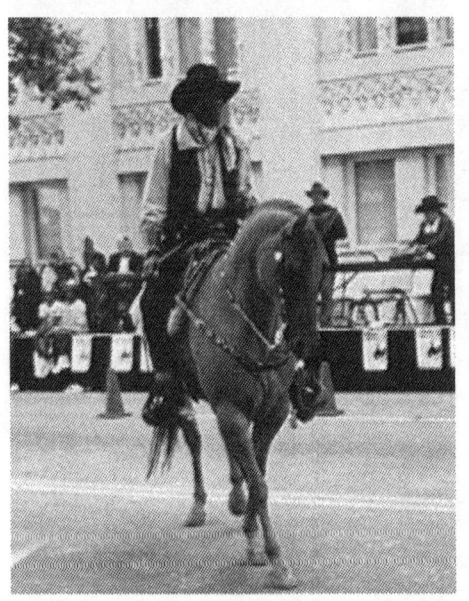

or serving in the owner's house. Many times we were shown walking or running. Most of the slaves performed hard back-breaking work in the fields and in the shops. But there still was those large mansions to maintain, also someone had to tend and feed the animals. By working with the animals that meant a lot us rode instead of walked. In many instances we knew more about the animals than our slave owners. On my Grand-father's farm many times my cousins would ride the horses. My Aunt Tippy (Mary Hardy, my father's younger sister) loved to ride the horses. Our image that we see portrayed today is one that was created by white historians and writers. Most people think of Blacks as people (heathens) who ran through the jungle half naked, killing off everything with spears (spear chuckers), but that isn't so.

I remember as a child my father regularly received newspapers from Nigeria, I was fascinated with the tall buildings, reading the news and advertisements (I learned something about other Blacks outside of America by reading the foreign newspapers he received). It was a big change from what I saw on television or at the movies, we weren't seen much except as servants, entertainers or criminals. It was rare if ever we saw a doctor, lawyer, or cowboy in a movie or television show who was Black, we always had to be rescued by a White or shown how to do something because we weren't intelligent enough. But, the Blacks in Africa were an educated group. They had their own education system in many

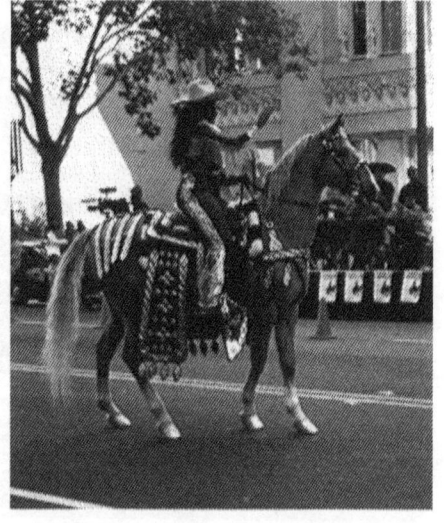

instances it was better than the Europeans or the Americans. A lot of the influences that brought about the changes in the African (Black) society was the coming of the Europeans and White Americans; we see the result of that today. They were farmers, cattlemen, warriors, artisans and politicians. These people were in constant motion; not just by foot, many of these tribes were nomads. The main mode of transportation was either camels or horses. So looking at our American history becoming Black horsemen and cattlemen was a natural move.

We weren't sheriffs fighting the bad guys and saving the damsels in distress. Black cowboys were working ranches and driving cattle long before many whites. A lot of these black cowboys and their families were free men not slaves. Black Cowboys took care of ranches, drove cattle, broke horses, and participated in Rodeos. The most famous Black rodeo star is Bill Pickett who is responsible for developing the art of bulldogging.

Thousands of Blacks moved to the west and mid-west after the Civil War, homesteading land and building homes and businesses for themselves and their families. As you go through the west today you will find Black ranchers and their cowboys still working hard. Enjoying what they do.

In keeping with the spirit of the Black Cowboys the Black Cowboys Associations for the past 23 years has sponsored a Black Cowboys parade in Oakland California. This year's parade was really nice. I took my grandchildren with me so that they could see the parade and some black history. Also participating in the parade was the Northern California Black Horseman Association. Let's not forget the women, there were plenty of Cowgirls. Did they leave the kids at home? NO! The kids rode their own horses or rode with their parents. The City of Hayward host the Black Cowboy rodeo. Both events have full support of the community. After the parade everyone has a chance to meet the cowboys and their horses. The rodeo is exciting because there are grownups and kids participating.

ALWAYS STRIVING TO IMPROVE

Being a person who has lived in many places and seen many things I've seen why people want to strive to improve. I've been in houses where there was no running water, or electricity. I've seen hungry kids fighting with the dog over the dog food. I been in villages and towns where the only

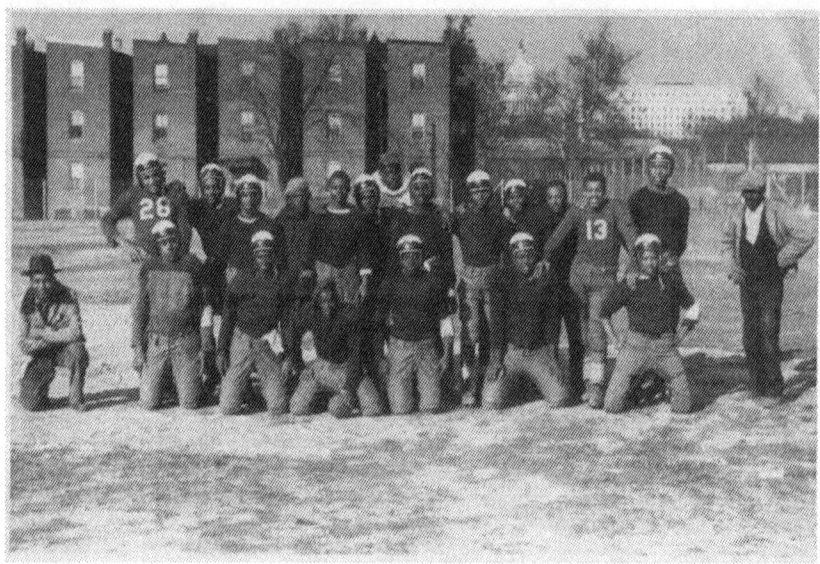

place you could get water was the central fountain and the oven for cooking was outside next to the toilet and chicken house. I've seen the one room school house my mother attended. And many times I saw her feed families that had been put out of their homes for non-payment of rent and all their possessions set on the street. Where jobs to Blacks were limited mostly to certain domestic, manual labor, and clerical areas. Many times this wasn't law but things encourage by the legal system. In an effort to improve I've found that many time you must confront the system, other social groups, family, friends and sometimes yourself. In an effort to create

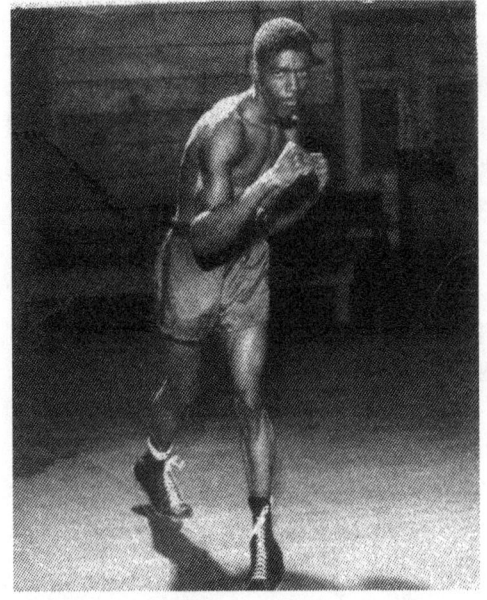

change people become upset because you will affect their status. Improving requires both a physical and mental change on everyones part. Remember striving to improve is a necessity not a gift.

Many times in an effort to improve you must use these past experiences as references to why you want to change, because there is no reason why you have to accept your present situation or condition.

Like any other migrant group in America, Blacks have always strived to get ahead. Leaving harsh environments to find something better. What do you consider harsh environments. Many of us Blacks see harsh as poor jobs, crowded schools, defacto segregation, weather, crime and etc. Many of our grandparents left area such as the south for many of these reasons including lynching. Mental, physical and financial growth was impossible because whites controlled everything. Even our education was controlled, many cities issued us blacks second rate or out-dated books. Our Black colleges picked up the slack but many saw educated Blacks as flukes instead of the norm. That attitude still exist today. Many Blacks migrated to California. They came by car, bus, or train. Many came to California during the Second World War. The economy was booming and there was plenty of jobs. And with those jobs was a man-power shorted. I asked one Black how his family came to California and he told me of how a white came to the town where he lived asking if anyone wanted to work and if so the company he worked for would pay for a one-way ticket for the family. His family migrated to California to work in the shipyards. Many of the jobs available to Blacks were in shipbuilding or Government Facilities.

Another Black who migrated to California was my Father-in-Law. He came to California first as a sailor in the Navy. Having completed his enlistment he went back to Beaumont Texas where he was married and later with his family and his mother and his sisters and brothers moved to California. While in Texas him and his brother played baseball in the Negro baseball league. Him

and his brother W.C Reed played for the Beaumont Athletics. After leaving Texas the family first stopped in Los Angeles where his mother worked as a maid. They eventually moved to Oakland California where he fought as a professional boxers under the name of Curtis JIGGS Reed. He eventually got a job as a aircraft mechanic at the Alameda Naval Air Station. A job he held until his retirement. Many of the older blacks had a can-do attitude and weren't afraid of challenges or competition. Many of our younger blacks today aren't or won't meet the challenges of today willing to go along as long as they get a little bit forgetting that a little bit is the same as nothing.

DISCRIMINATION STILL LINGER

Discrimination still lingers here America and the evidence is here in proposition 209. Why do you want to get rid of Affirmative Action in the government sector unless you don't like the idea of dealing with minorities. If it wasn't for affirmative Action you whites would still be living in your Ivory Tower looking over your dominion. To get back some of your god type attitude you use prop. 209 as the key.

Some of you Asians and Hispanics who support this proposition are even bigger fools. Look at your history. Blacks didn't deprive you of anything, whites did. Blacks had nothing to deprive you of. We didn't work you to death building railroads across country. We didn't encourage you to come to this country illegally to work and after you've completed your task create laws to deport you. How many of you Blacks have become indifferent saying I've got mines why worry about you. We blacks fought hard to get where we're at today. It was mostly due to laws like Affirmative Action. We fought for equal pay, access to housing, transportation and most important equal access to the Law. Now attempts are being made to slowly take those rights away. In order to grow you can't depend on the Welfare System, you can't depend on Drugs the only end there is Jail or death in many areas drugs have been the destruction of Communities. You must learn to make the system work if you want growth. You must learn to work in the system to make it work. A good way to start is that you must vote. Don't tell me I'm wrong because how did prop. 209 pass. It was because a lot of blacks didn't vote how foolish are we. After coming this far we've now allowed people to ease back to being their same old evil negative self.

Where does voting start? It's starts in your local area. If you want to make a change you must first start with your local officials. This means your Mayor, Councilman, City manager and all those commissioner seats. You must develop political clout. Remember everything starts with the City Council and that means everything including approval of funds. Politics start locally and work up to the National level.

By not voting you're actually voting for people you don't like or trust. Just think why you should vote you're voting for access to government, opportunity. Don't you want better schools, medical facilities, safer public transportation, better public housing? The list can go on and on, but the decision is up to you. Are you part of the crowd that's always complaining but when it's time for action you pass the responsibility on to someone else and when things don't work out you say that no-one is looking out for you. The truth is that the opposition knows you better than you know yourself and they depend on your inactivity to help them. This is how Prop 209 got through due to voters complacence. If you want to see positive change, **VOTE**.

We were taken out of slavery and because of neglect and foolishness we're allowing ourselves to slide back into a negative similar type situation. One of my readers gave me an article printed in the Open forum. She wanted me to read it because it showed the deterioration of the black family do to drug. The writer spoke of a high school friend that she knew well in school. And now he's in jail for dealing drugs. When asked about his family he explains to her that he was raised by his grandmother, his mother is a drug addict, his father who he seldom saw was just sentenced to 53 years to life. His reason for dealing drugs was the money, money represented power and there you could buy anything and as a youngster he saw all this on TV. What a sense of false reality we as a people are picking up. And it's reflected in our youth. We face discrimination, drugs and it seems like a lot of people are trying to tell us it's alright to support crime and you should feel fine looking down on yourself and being treated second class.

AFFIRMATIVE ACTION TAKES NEW BLOW

Federal Judge Lynn N. Hughes ruled that white male members of the Houston Texas Contractors Association had unfairly lost business because of Metro Affirmative Action Program. Metro's program was setup to give Woman and Minority own business 21% of the contracts. The Judge said we do not accept the concept that a person is responsible for what others of her race, town, profession, or politics may have done.

Reading this article in the paper is upsetting. What's being said is that it's alright for White contractors and business to deprive us blacks of business based mainly on our color but if White business lose money due to competition with us then we are wrong because now we are depriving him of business due to unfair competition. It appears to me that many white males feel that because of their color they should automatically be given contracts. Something I've noticed in this suit is that the Judge was supposed to be ruling for White Males but in her ruling she spoke as if the case was dealing with women. I wonder if she really looked at this suit. Or was it a political move for her. For us small black businesses it's harder because we depend on the larger businesses which are mostly White. Most of them don't want to use us and with these laws of requirement being removed that means we Blacks are back at square one. If the law says we minorities should receive 21% of the contracts and everyone else should get 79% how are we treating whites unfairly unless they believe that they as a group should receive all 100%.

If all these cases against Affirmative Action were looked at fairly the rulings would always be in favor of Affirmative Action. What the Whites are saying is that they don't want blacks or minorities to have any positions, jobs or contracts. And if any are to be given out it is of their (Whites) choosing. And their intentions are not to give out any. They want to go back to the good ole boy system of awarding contracts and jobs. One suit pending is where a White female professor is upset because she was fired and not the equally qualified Black. All this goes back to the old standard of Blacks are the last to be hired and the first to be fired.

In our struggle to improve we find that whites try even harder to resist change. A white youth in Denver, Colorado shot a Black man because he felt that the Black man didn't belong. In Texas some White men dragged a Black man to death behind their truck. Whites are continually struggling to remove Affirmation Action. Racial strife is still going on in America. Whites are still teaching racial hatred. We Blacks have been given full equal rights but, even with the passing of legislation we're still fighting battles in the court room and on the street. Now that Blacks are out in the marketplace Whites are complaining, because now they must compete against us as equals and in many cases they find that we are better qualified. Now they complain because jobs they felt were guaranteed are now going to the better qualified blacks; many of them find this insulting. How quickly people forget? Blacks attend the same schools as they do, go through the same training, fight the same wars and pay taxes. We Blacks have the same wants and desires as them. Most of us aren't on Welfare, we aren't criminals, thieves, drug addicts, or hookers. So quit trying to stereotype us. Basically, Whites are afraid of competition, because now their competing against the world community and the competition at home is getting tougher. What you must realize is that we're trying to work with you and for things to move forward we must work on an equal and balanced foundation. This thing of a divided country is only for fools! For this country to survive everyone must work together. Understand one thing, this country was built on everyones blood, sweat and tears. So, you Whites quit trying to act as if you alone built this country. We must focus on our similarities instead of our differences; anything else is divisive (it only keeps us apart). The chains of Slavery was taken off BLACKS over 100 years ago, *now we must break those mental chains of slavery.*

NEWS FLASH

Negroes Allowed to Join Navy

DEPARTMENT OF THE NAVY—NAVAL HISTORICAL CENTER
901 M STREET SE—WASHINGTON NAVY YARD
WASHINGTON DC 20374-5060

Navy Department Press Release: Navy to Accept Negroes for General Service

For release following Secretary of the Navy's press conference, Tuesday, April 7, 1942

The Navy Department today announced that Negro volunteers will be accepted for enlistment for general service in the reserve components of the U.S. Navy, the U.S. Marine Corps, and the U.S. Coast Guard.

All ratings in those three branches of the Naval Service will be opened to them and recruiting is to be begun as soon as a suitable training station is established. A public announcement will be made when actual recruiting gets under way.

In making this announcement officials stated that the same physical and mental entrance standards required of all Navy personnel is to be required of Negroes.

It was added when Negro sailors are to be utilized for duty in District craft of various kind, in maritime activities around shore establishments, in Navy Yards, and in the Navy's new construction crews and companies which will be employed in developing bases outside the United States' continental limits.

Recruiting of Negroes for service in the Messman Branch is to continue without change or interruption.

Source: Document reproduced in MacGregor, Morris J. and Bernard C. Nalty. *Blacks in the United States Armed Forces: Basic Documents.* vol.6. Wilmington DE: Scholarly Resources, 1977, p. 103.

ABOUT THE MILITARY

Ships

During my career in the military I did a lot of growing-up. You had to work long hours sometimes under extreme conditioner and for little pay. My first ship a Aircraft Carrier the USS Midway. To me it was huge with its 8 boilers and 4 engines4 generator room,8 generators (for electricity), during a cruise to Vietnam we had a crew of about 5,000 and 100 planes(fighters, bomber, reconnaissance planes and helo's for rescue).Next I was transferred to one of the smallest ship USS CREE ATF 84 a fleet tug. It was part of Service Pacific Fleet operating out of San Diego, California. She serviced with such Fleet tugs as the USS APACHE, USS TAWASA., USS SIOUX, USS UTE and the list goes on. Many of these tugs actually saw combat during the Second World, Korea, and Vietnam. Although these ships were tugs, they were outfitted with weapons for combat. The Cree was about 100 feet long with its main defense being one 3" gun. The ship had a range of 13000 miles. We had a hundred man crew. The ship was 2/3 engineroom and the fuel tank was from the engine room to underneath crews berthing. When the weather became hot the fuel in the tanks would expand and leak into the berthing compartments where you slept. You could slide across the deck there was so much oil. The ship was diesel electric which means that engineering was mostly Engine repairman and Electricians. Its main power plant was 4 huge diesel engines. Even with duties like towing targets (most of the time ships fired at us instead of the target),At sea rescue, towing ships and vessel along the west coast from South America to Alaska ,and almost getting sucked under ships during transfer and refueling underway, it was good duty. We went to South America, Alaska, Japan, Taiwan and Vietnam.

Another ship I enjoyed serving on was the USS PAGE FFG 5 home-ported Athens Greece. That was one fascinating ship. It was a Fast Frigate with missiles. It had one engineroom and one fireroom (2 boilers). It was the first ship I had been on with 1200 lb, 920 degree superheated steam system. The steam was so hot it could cut you in half with just a pin hole leak. The most unusual part was that the boilers had superchargers which meant you could get underway quick. We serve in Lebanon, Israel and we were there for the Greece/Turkey crisis.

I was one of the original crew-members when the ship was transferred from Newport, Rhode Island to Athens, Greece as part of Destroyer Squadron 12. Destroyer Squadron 12 consisted of 6 ships USS Sampson DDG-10, USS Barry DD-933, USS Manley DD-941, USS Veerland FF-1068, USS Wood DD-715, and the USS Page FFG-5, with the Guided Missile Destroyer Sampson acting as the squadrons flag ship. For my family that was exciting because the Navy placed them on a Amphibious Assault ship and transported them to Greece. They were at sea 2 weeks. The ship stopped in South Carolina, Spain, Italy and finally Greece.

The Guided Missile Cruiser USS BIDDLE CG 34 was another ship I enjoyed. We only had 12 electricians but everyone was good. My sons went on an overnight cruises and they got a chance to see the guns fire and missiles launched. The ship even went to Constanta, Romania in the Soviet Union. This was before the fall of the Soviet Union, we went there with the Soviet fleet. Because Destroyers and Cruisers are always operating with Carriers there are always hazards. On November 22 1975 the USS BELKNAP CG 26 sister ship to the BIDDLE was run over by the carrier USS KENNEDY CVA 67 it wasn't sunk but the bridge and superstructure was destroyed and everyone there was killed. Fuel pipes ruptured on the carrier and dumping fuel down the smoke stacks and into the fireroom of the BELKNAP and the fire and 1200 lbs of steam killed a lot of sailors in engineering. The fire was so hot that the part of the ships super structure melted around some of the sailors instantly killing them. Ironically the Destroyer that came to the BELKNAPS aid was struck by the same carrier the next day and was so badly damaged that it had to be decommissioned. Some of the survivors from the BELKNAP were later transferred to the BIDDLE for duty.

BLACK SAILORS

My time in the Navy was fascinating. Blacks have serviced in the Navy for years. Before World War Two we serviced on ships as Stewards, Commissaryman(cooks), and Ship Serviceman (These job titles have all been changed). These were the people that cooked the crews and the officers meals, they operated the ships laundry, they cut the officers hair, and they cleaned the officers quarters. Although they weren't allowed to work in other trades they still had to handle ammunition, help clean boilers, or maintain those then wooden ship decks sometimes as a collateral duty and sometimes as a punishment . It wasn't until April 7, 1942 that we were officially allowed to work in other fields(Boatswains Mate, Gunners Mate, Boiler Technician, and Machinist Mates . We gradually begin to work in other fields such as aircraft and submarines Because of segregation during the Second World War many Blacks sailors often served on ships operated by an all Black crew. You saw many whites serving on Submarines, but a lot of Blacks died on those sunken ships during the second World War. It wasn't until the sixties and seventies that we were eventually allowed to work in any field. Coming out of high school and into the Navy was a big change for me. I entered the Navy at a time when the Navy was starting to show change. Integration was in full swing and ship design was changing. There was construction of super guided missile cruisers like the Columbus CG 12, and Chicago CG 11. Unlike missile carrying ships of today that have one or two missile launchers these had four and carried almost 200 missiles including weapons for anti-submarine warfare. This meant they could confront many targets at one time. These ships were as high and almost as long as a Aircraft carrier, I smile because these were great war ships. For me as a Black here was true opportunity. During my time in the Navy I learned responsibility, to look at things with an open mind. There I was taught to be creative and have

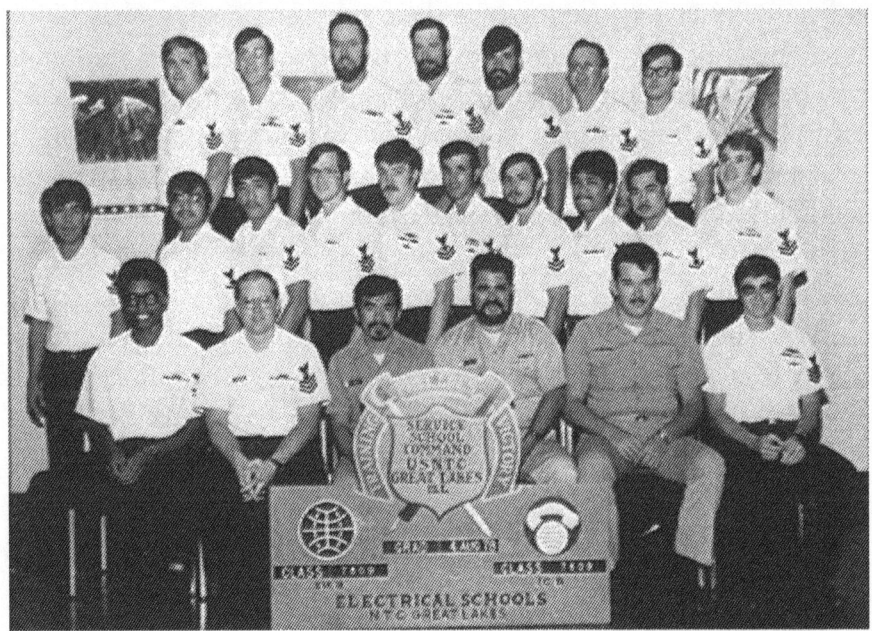

imagination. As an engineer you learn that equipment had to be working no matter what. I was awakened many times in the middle of the night because we electricians had to pull a pump motor or ventilation motor. While on the Midway CVA-41 there was a fire in #4 Switchboard room, after the damage control party had put the fire out we electricians worked around clock to get everything working. Blacks were in the middle of everything. I still remember the smell of black crude oil which was used for fuel. A lot of the Blacks were machinist mates or boiler technicians working in extreme heat and unbearable conditions. I remember on many occasions working in knee deep water repairing a motor to get a pump back on line. As an engineer you learn quickly that when you're at sea you must repair equipment immediately because you have no-one to make repairs because you are out there by yourself . In the movies you always saw these clean sailors, no one spoke of those sailors in engineering that kept the ship running and when you did see someone they were white. A lot of Blacks in engineering lost their lives on those sunken ships. Although we Blacks on ships were few we were everywhere. You found many Blacks in trades that were extremely dirty or skills most whites didn't want. Blacks in the Boatswains Mate field spent many hours sitting in boatswains chairs draped over the side of ships chipping and painting the ships hull and anchor. We also worked on aircraft, in communications, in weapons, and nuclear fields. We spent long periods of time in navy schools enhancing our skills. Many times I found myself as the only Black in a class. These weren't simple classes but strict educational classes where military discipline was enforced. My first Black division officer was Lt. Lewis he was our Electrical division officer on the cruiser Biddle CG-34. He was later transferred to the Nuclear Power cruiser Long Beach CGN-9. He was a very fine officer.

Midway Island, yes we were there. Blacks were there working on aircraft. When you think of aircraft remember the people that worked on them. They maintain the engines, repaired structural damage with their main responsibility being to keep those planes flying. My friend Eugene Edwards was one those assigned to a fighter squadron out of Texas that was attached to Midway Island and later Japan and Carrier duty in the Mediterranean. Gene entered the Navy an airman apprentice and left as a Second Class Petty Officer working on everything from prop driven to jet aircraft. The navy for Blacks in the 40's and 50's was hard, because we were limited to certain fields. Advancement was even worse, because for whites the sky was the limit but for blacks as high as most went was Second Class Petty Officer. I talked to a Black senior who had served on Navy ships during the 50's and he told me that when he made 3rd class

Petty officer there was only a selected number of ships he could serve on because the Whites didn't want Blacks telling them what to do. Most of the changes for Blacks came during the 60's and 70's. But many of these changes came after riots and fights between whites and Blacks on and off many ships. Because of those changes I retired as a Chief Petty Officer with 21 years service and my position was ship superintendent.

SECRETS-Blacks kept secrets very well. If information on ships movement or weapons got out it was usually due to someone White and if you check the newspapers today you fine that it still holds true. So don't believe that story about us Blacks talking too much.

HAVING SERVED THIS COUNTRY WELL, BLACKS HAVE EARNED THE RIGHTS, LIBERTY AND RESPECT THAT TODAY THEY MUST DEMAND

Advancing Upward

During my time in the Navy, one of the most important things to me was advancements. With advancement came privileges and responsibilities and the best part was higher pay. To me advancement was important because I saw many Blacks retire as E-5 and this was the norm and I wanted to go higher. Advancing to Chief Petty Officer E-7 was the hardest accomplishment in my career. I had taken the Chief examination four times and passed (test are given once a year) and was never selected by the Bureau of Personnel in Washington for advancement. Upset and angry I sort counseling from Master Chief Blake a Black. Why did I seek counsel from him, I felt I would get real information from him than his white counter part. I went to his office and he talk to me for an hour and when he finish talking I was really hyped. Advancement to E-7 isn't easy because not only do you have to meet job plus educational requirements, because of the competitiveness I found that you must do things to set yourself apart from the crowd. After talking to the Master Chief, I enrolled in more Navy schools and college classes, became a counselor and started taking on more responsibility and a year and a half later I was notified of advancement.

This was the high point in my Navy career. This is when your uniform changed from dungaree to khaki. Even after notification of my advancement from E-6 to E-7 (CHIEF PETTY OFFICER) advancing wasn't going to be easy. Once notified of your advancement to chief petty officer by the Bureau of Personnel in Washington, D.C. your greatest test is the chief initiation, which starts immediately, and it lasts about a month. Everyone advancing to Chief goes through the initiation (male and female). I was excited about advancement and the anticipation about the initiation had me scared because there wasn't a clue of what the chiefs had planned. At the command where I was station there was about 10 of us prospective chiefs and we had to march every day into the chiefs mess hall like ducks (that included the quacking). Whenever we ate in the Chiefs mess we had to eat what the chiefs fixed for us and we weren't allowed to sit in chairs. One of their favorite things was an egg in tomato juice, and it didn't taste too bad. Sometimes someone would put a cigarette out in your food. No, you didn't have to eat the cigarette. In the CPO mess we would be given daily assignments and they had to be done or we would be fined. Each of us were assigned an additional 10 tasks to do before advancement day. Some of these things seemed impossible, especially when you're stationed on a large ship, I was stationed on a repair ship. Once assigned these tasks you learn to use research, imagination and just maintain a can-do attitude to accomplish your goals. Some of the items I had to get,

- A quart jar of fresh watermelon seeds
- 10lbs of fresh horse manure
- A snake
- Two frogs
- An autographed G-string from a GO-GO dancer

I got everything (smile), but I spent half a day at a horse ranch. The kids and I were out in woods at night looking for frogs and snakes. I spent some time with a watermelon grower learning about watermelons. And the G-string was custom made by my wife and I went to one of the local clubs and a dancer signed it. One of the guys had to get an autograph from MISS BLACK VIRGINIA, yes, he got the autograph and like a lot of us he had to do his homework. Everyone was given a book that you were required to have all the chiefs sign and you were told not to lose it, the Chiefs put a rope or heavy chain through it and you wore it all the time, because losing it meant a fine. Ships Company got one of the books and took it to the rifle range and shot it to pieces and when it was returned it looked like a rag.

The high point of the advancement to CPO was advancement day. Your work day started at five o'clock A.M. and you worked in the CPO mess until about 9:00 A.M. you were then taken to the base where the advancement ceremony was to take place. Once you arrived, you changed into a costume selected by the chiefs assigned to you. I won't describe my costume except to say I had to wear high heel shoes. After arriving you were brought before a judge. While waiting to see the judge the chiefs would think of something for you to do. One of their favorite jokes was giving you an egg and telling you to hold it in your mouth until they returned and they would take forever to come. Usually they would return when it was time for you to meet the judge. Here I was charged with something and I argued with the judge like crazy, I was even given a lawyer that was usually a junior officer and the complete thing was a setup so I lost. If your lawyer defended you, he received the same fate as you, so he didn't say much. I was found guilty and placed in a coffin, once in the coffin it was closed and locked. Next it was filled with food, beer and liquor and I stayed there for about 10 minutes, when I was let out of the box I smelled terrible.

After the initiation all of us prospective chiefs cleaned up and assembled for the advancement ceremony, there the Judge explains its purpose, next your commanding officer talks to you, and finally someone of your choosing pins on your anchors, for me it was my wife. Unlike other enlisted that wear stripes on the left arm of their uniform, Chiefs wear collar devises shaped as anchors. All of us new chiefs were sharp because this was the proudest point of our career. What the initiation taught you was that you would be assigned difficult tasks some seemingly impossible but with imagination and initiative you can accomplish your goal.

Sometimes you are going to lose through no fault of your own, but you are not to let these problems get you down; just press on and still walk with pride.

Black Sailors Today

Black sailors today serve on all Navy ships, starting with nuclear powered submarines to Aircraft carriers. I had the opportunity to sail on the repair ship U.S.S. Cape Cod AD-43 with my youngest son. My wife and I flew to Hawaii where I met the ship, and I sailed with son from Hawaii to San Diego, it was a very informative cruise. I had the opportunity to see the ship from the bridge to engineering. I also met the Captain and Executive Officer. The ship had a crew of about 1000 sailors, men and women. It had the capacity to repair any ship afloat. My son was assigned as a welder. During the two week trip I tried to meet and talk to everyone. My son acted as my tour guide and he took me everywhere. The trip was called a tiger cruise. In today's Navy you see a lot of new changes. My son took me into engineering where there is a lot of machinery all maintain by the ships crew. We went up to computer room that keeps track of everything and everybody. They didn't have this on ships when I was sailor. I went to the Television studio and what a setup. Then he took me down to the Repair Department. Here you see modern equipment to repair all types of equipment you name it and these people can repair it. Don't forget those cooks because they put together some outstanding meals. Times have really changed for the Navy because now many of your Black sailors aren't High School Graduates but college students with 2 or more years of college and that's officer and enlisted.

MEMORIES

Have you ever looked back on your past? You can't change your past, but you can use those experiences to change your future for the better. I remember one of the first cars my wife and I bought, it was a 3 cylinder Saab we bought for $25.00. Before we could even drive it we had to dig it out from a pile of leaves and dirt. Next we had to install a new floorboard and replace the seats because everything had rotted. Next the amazement of seeing the window wipers blow off in the rain. It sounded like a lawn mower with a top speed of 70 miles per hour. I smile fondly when I think of my trip to Hawaii with my wife to meet the ship my son was serving on. After meeting the ship I had the opportunity to spend two weeks on the ship with him from Hawaii to San Diego California. Do you remember your childhood? As a Black I've found many people to day have a distorted view of the black community or our past in general. Today the image viewed by many is the distorted picture created by the media (newspapers and television). For many of us raised in Black communities in the 40's, 50's and early 60's life was totally different. I remember a community where you were taught self worth and respect for others. Where family, education, working, church, and community were important.

Some of the people that had a strong influence on my life with positive teaching and examples were my mother's parents, Yelly and Laura Warren (born 1888 and 1890 respectively). My father's parents Alexander Piner of Chestertown Maryland, and Carrie Fisher of Washington D.C. died before I was born. My grandparents were part of that first generation after the end of slavery; they were part of a brave new world. My grandfather was a quiet man who worked hard and didn't smoke or drink. Here was a

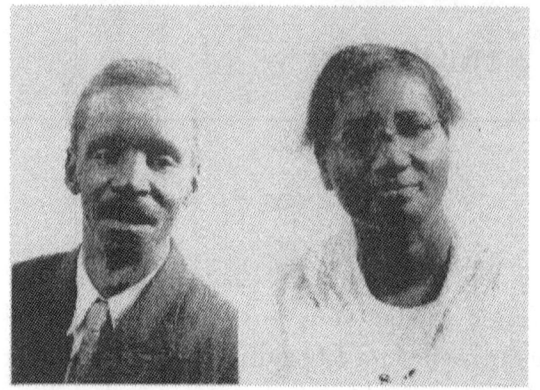

man with only a third grade education who built one of the largest farms in his area, over 200 acres. Although a short person about 5'6", to me he was a big man. I remember standing in a chair next to him watching with fascination as he shaved in front of the kitchen mirror. While watching him hitch animals to the different pieces of equipment I would imagine myself being able to handle animals as gently as him. I saw him angry only once and that was when some hawks attempted to take some of his chickens. You never forgot that incident because he came running out of the house with shotgun firing away.

My grandmother was the disciplinarian of the family. She taught me a valuable lesson, if you don't work you don't eat. One day she told me to do some work and trying to be smart, I said no. At dinnertime instead of allowing me to eat she sent me to bed and I cried all night, but I never again said no to any work. This wasn't a woman who went to parties, but a woman with high moral values who stood with her husband and family. My grandmother was a tall, proud woman with neatly braided hair and while washing cloths, working in her garden, or cooking she always wore those neat cotton house dresses. On Sundays the women would straighten my grandmothers hair and she wore her Sunday best. My grandparent's lives weren't boring, but interesting. I remember my mother showing me with pride one of the houses my grandparents lived in with their children while building their main house. The house was really a stable, which housed the work animals. The stable now long gone was demolished and the well for water now filled in after a new stable was built my grandparent's kitchen and living area was on the first floor, the animals were located in the stable area in the front, and everyone slept on the second floor where the hay was stored. These people possess little education, but they had the determination to grow and build, and they passed these values onto the younger generations.

My grandparents lived in the Black farm community of Hill Top, Maryland. Here was a small, modest community of farmers and trades-man. A community where half the families was related, aunts, uncles and cousins everywhere and that included great-aunts and great-uncles. The center of all social activity was the church, Zion Baptist. Behind the church was the one room school building everyone attended, in fact it was the same school my mother attended in the 30's. This was a community that had only one store, which also acted as the Post Office and the gas station. I never forgot that two lane blacktop that served as the main road with its neatly maintained farm houses and manicured lawns on each side, and the sight of farmers working their fields of corn, tobacco, and later peanuts. There was the picking of apples, peaches, plums, black berries, and blue berries which all the kids in the family picked during the summer and the women canned, getting ready for winter. I was always getting stung by bee's and hornets or scratched by briers while picking berries. I remember my cousins and I knocking down a bee's nest while picking pears and those angry bee's had us running for dear life. There was also the killing of hogs, which was butchered, smoked and cured and stored in the smokehouse. Cows were strictly for dairy products.

Living with my grandparents was a fun period in my life. When I was old enough to go to school I stayed with my parents in Washington, D.C., and during the summer I would live with my grandparents. I didn't feel lonesome living with my grandparents because there were so many kids in the family. There were aunts, uncles, and cousins and we were all close in age. There was Sam, James Jr., Yancey Jr., John Jr. and me Warren Jr., Roger Lee, Richard, Jonathan, Hazel, Hilda, Laverne, Christine, Rachel,

Madeline, Tippy(Mary), Joann, Joan, Judy and Elnore. My Uncle Sam acted more like a older brother and my Aunt Christine acted more like an older sister, there was only a four or five year difference in our ages. At one time there were so many kids staying with my grandparents that there was four or five of us boys sleeping in one bed. And the older girls had the same problem. I remember the girls always arguing about whose wearing whose cloths. At that time you didn't have central heating. There was a wood burning stove for heating in every room for a total of seven and in cold weather my grandmother kept the fires burning in all of them. The largest stove was in the kitchen for cooking and making hot water. There was no running water all our water came from a well, this meant there was no toilet in the bathroom, you had a night bucket and every bedroom had a wash basin for freshening up. Even without the conveniences that everyone is accustomed to today you still felt comfortable.

There was excitement living on the farm. I remember when the day started you always got up early, but I could never get up earlier than my grandparents. They would get up around five o'clock lighting fires in the stoves for heating and cooking, and planning their day. By the time all of us kids got up my grandmother and all the women and the older girls were up and cooking. We all ate as a family at one huge table and if that table was full some of us ate at the table in the kitchen. There were so many of us kids at the table that instead of using chairs my grandfather built benches. One of the things I enjoyed at breakfast was hot buttered biscuits dipped in King syrup. King was the brand name and it had a special taste almost like honey.

Everyone had something to do from feeding the animals to cutting wood. I always remember that woodpile because at the start of winter my grandfather and the men would bring in fresh wood and that pile looked like it was 15 to 20 feet high. The older boys would go to the stable get the horses and hitch them to the wagons. On my Grandfather's farm I saw the change from farm animals, to tractors and other machinery such as milling machines for grinding grain. My grandfather coordinated the use of horses and tractors for certain tasks. Horses were used to pull large rakes for gathering hay and cutters for cutting corn and other crops. The tractor was used with equipment that didn't need an attendant. After working the

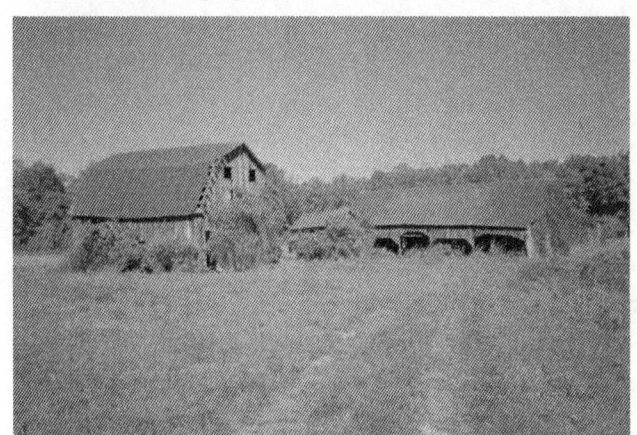

horses we kids would take them to the water trough and then to the stable for feeding. Because the water trough was next to the rear door of the house sometimes things would get exciting while giving the horses water, because the horses would start fighting and everyone would run into the house including the animals. Eventually my grandfather closed in the porches because my grandmother was tired of chasing animals out of the kitchen.

A major event on the farm was the harvesting of tobacco. To harvest tobacco we used horse drawn wagons. First my grandfather would top the tobacco, that's breaking the flowers on the top of the plant. Next my grandfather and the older boys would cut the tobacco, the rest of the grownups and all of us kids would spear the tobacco and place it on the wagon. (Spearing—staffs with a sharp metal point, which is driven through the stalk of the Plant in preparation for hanging in the barns for curing). The spear is about 6' long and you put stalks of tobacco on them until you only have only enough room for your hands then you would load the tobacco on wagons. Once the wagon was loaded we took the tobacco to the barns for aging and curing. Although this was exciting work I did have one scary moment and that was when I lost my balance while riding a wagon load of tobacco to the barn, falling off, and rolled under the wagon. One of the wagons metal wheels ran over my toes cutting them. My cousins rushed me to my grandmother and she band-aged my foot and had me back working and playing again. My foot was cut so easily because like all the kids I wasn't wearing any shoes. My grand-father had 3 barns with the largest being about 3 stories. I saw working in them as scary work because they were very big places with large double doors front and rear for your wagons access and exit. When you started work all you had to walk on were rafters. There were no floors just the ground. But, while working high above hanging tobacco my cousins walked those rafters like trapeze artist. You put the spears of tobacco between rafters with their stalks of tobacco leaves hanging down. A stalk of tobacco would be about 4' tall, and with everyone working you fill the barns from the roof down to about a foot from the ground, and not a space would be missed. The tobacco would be hung all the way to the barn doors then the barns would be closed. You always remembered that sweet pleasant smell of the tobacco plants. It's amazing how with all that tobacco no one smoked cigarettes and this I believe was because of their religion teaching.

While everyone was working, the women would be cooking. To let everyone know when it was time to eat my grandmother would signal by using the car horn. I'll always remember those meals because everything was fresh or home canned, very little was bought from the store the corn meal for bread was produced by the family mill. Because the family was large, everything was served on platters and I didn't want to miss a meal.

Sundays was the big day, because that was when members of the family living in the county would eat dinner at my grandparent's home. There was no cooking, because everything was prepared on Saturday. There would be so many at the house that three tables would be setup. I remember my father assembling all the elders together for the taking of pictures. What a crowd, there was my grandparents, great-aunt Mamie, great-aunt Katie, great-uncle Simms and great-uncle Sunn and all their kids. All of us kids after eating would play all types of games. I remember games such as Badminton, Hide and Seek, Baseball, and checkers. The really tough game was Hide and Seek because you had so many places to hide, that included under the house, in the hedges, and in some of the small fields close by. Although there wasn't any television I remember spending evenings sitting in the sitting room trying to read the older kids school books.

During the break in the farming season my grandfather and uncles would go hunting, fishing, or crabbing and when they returned home all of us kids would anxiously wait to see what they had and what ever they brought home we help to clean. My grandfather was also a master carpenter and I saw many of the buildings he constructed withstand some violent storms and the test of time.

Living with my grandparents, I remember running barefoot through the fields. After my grandfather plowed his fields, we kids would take the sod and build African style huts, which we used for play. And when it rained you remembered the massage like feel of mud between the toes. You learn to try new things, I was taught to eat certain wild plants and to use the bark off certain trees to make tea. I remember looking in amazement at my aunt's milking cows and afterwards all of us churning butter in the kitchen. It was fascinating watching my grandfather and all the older boys grinding the corn at the milling machine in the garage. And don't forget the animals, the smell of chickens, pigs, horses, cows, and turkeys.

To visit my grandparent farm was always an enjoyable adventure, riding the Trailway bus, picking watermelons in the watermelon patch. One of the most exciting times was when my grandparents would put all us smaller kids in that old forties Ford automobile, and they would take us into town with them where they would buy trays of baby chicks that they would later raise in the chicken house, and buy seedling plants in preparation for the next growing season. I never forgot the dogs Rags and Spot, they always seem to enjoy chasing me. Lets not forget those fresh eggs from the chicken house. Hearing my grandfathers tractor, watching him operate those different pieces of equipment and like kids everywhere when he went in the house I would sit on the equipment and imitate him. The farm though smaller is still in operation today, but managed by my Aunt

Madeline and her brothers Nathaniel and Yancey. Crops have changed and a pond has been added for ducks and geese with duck crossing signs being posted on the main road. The family as grown to well over 200 people and still growing, becoming as diversified as a small nation. In an ever-changing world many times we forget about those small positive times, always dwelling on those negative things that create bitterness and hate. Many of us forget to draw on those pleasant memories that help us smile during adverse times. But those pleasant memories you never forget because they spark your imagination encouraging you to want to do things, to build and to grow. As a Black and a cancer patient I find that now I face a double threat. Times and attitudes have change and many not for the better, but those positive memories are still there and now I must draw on those images to help me survive and recover. You want people to understand that you're not reminiscing or trying to relive your past, but you are drawing on those small positive memories using them to enhance or improve your future.

HOME

As a youth living with my grandparents was fun, but I still looked forward to being with parents Warren and Irene Fisher. We lived in various places in Washington D. C.. Our first house was a two bedroom alley house on Fenton Place in northwest Washington; when you stepped out the front door you were in the alley. After living in several places we finally moving into the projects known as Simms Drive. To my parents the projects were nice, the only problems with public housing was the use of kerosene for heating and cooking, everyone in the projects shared a party phone line and you had to walk over a mile to catch the bus. We eventually moved to the Barry Farms housing projects with central heating provided by a coal fired furnace. Here my father was always involved in some type of community activity. My sister Joann like my father was also active in community events I remember her going to dance classes and later in junior high school working as a volunteer red cross nurses aid in the

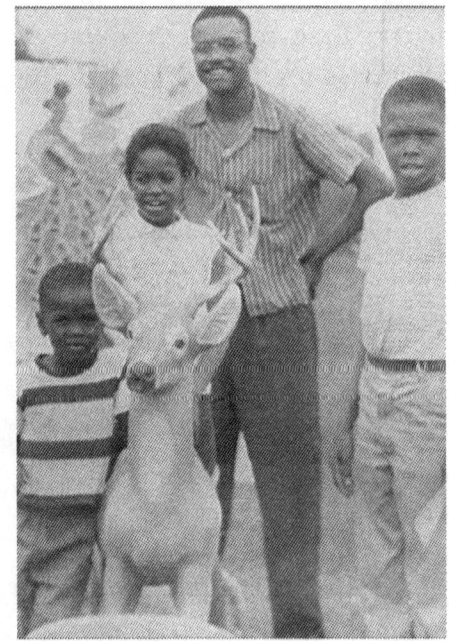

local hospitals. My mother a busy housewife was always helping people. If a family was put out on the street for non-payment of rent she would feed them, if a women was having a baby my mother and her sisters would get clothes and diapers for the new baby. She was always on the go doing something.

During the summer my father would always fine things to do or places to go. He would take my sister, brother and me on train trips to New York, Philadelphia, New Jersey, and Baltimore. We would go to the beach, and when the circus and carnival was in town my father would always take us. On those really hot days my father would stop at Fishermans Wharf and buy fresh blue crabs and bring them home and cook them in beer and his special seasoning. Eating those tastee crabs was a treat. To add a little excitement to everything, before cooking the crabs he would knock over the bag of crabs and we kids would be running everywhere trying to get away from claws. I remember when he and his friends would have their weekly card game sessions. To me this was exciting because I would be allowed to sip some of their beer. At night he entertained me with stories. He created toy construction kits (projects) for me to play with and I could call him at work any time.

I remember in my youth of seeing pictures of my father when he was in the Army, he served during World War II. His photo album was like looking at a big story book because of all the black soldiers; they were the best looking people in the world. 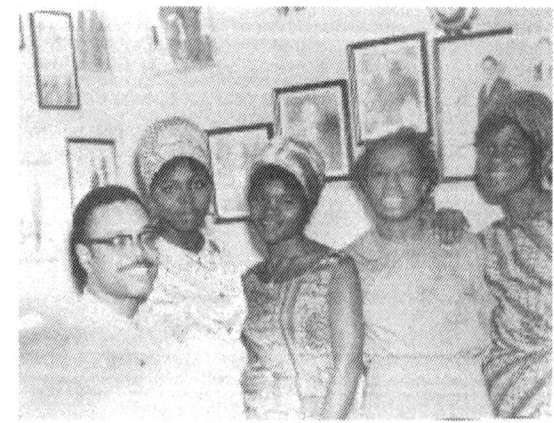 After coming out of the Army my father was always improving himself; trying to move up he went to school at night or took correspondent courses. Being a man of many languages his second language was French which he learned as a youth. Before it became politically correct my father had African family and friends stay at our home. Some were students and some were political figures. On many occasions he went on extended trips to Africa living in the local villages. With all this activity going on my mother was there to support him. I remember the African newspapers we always received and my native costume given to me when I became 18 years old. My father worked as a clerk in Civil Service for about twenty-five years and retired at the age of 55. I asked him why he retired and he

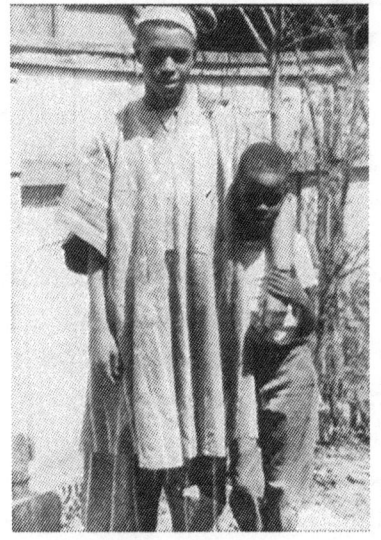

said he was tired of training whites and then seeing the whites he trained become his supervisor. He knew how the system worked and he played it well, but being Black he knew he would only rise so far (he had hit that glass ceiling). After retiring he maintained his interest in local politics, African affairs and writing. His main love was writing and photography, he wrote for many local black newspapers under the name of FABULOUS FISHER (FAB) a name he still use today.

My mother was always there helping my father with his many ideas. When she wasn't being a busy housekeeper and mother she was going to Night School and studying. Next to family her next love was the church, she took my sister, brother and I to church every Sunday, to prayer service on Friday and bible study on Tuesdays. With this ambition she became the churches Sunday School superintendent and eventually becoming a Lay Speaker. Because of my parents teachings and just watching them do things I knew I wanted to eventually own a business and be involved in activities.

TRAVELING THROUGH TIME

Traveling though time leaves pleasant memories. Living with my grandparent leaves pleasant memories. Memories are combination of everything. The closeness of the family. To me it's the smell and warmth of the wood stove. The sounds of the people cooking in the kitchen. The sounds and smell of farm animal. The taste of fresh vegetable grown in the family garden. The sounds of Christmas and the taste of Christmas sugar cookies and candies. The smell of a fresh cut Christmas tree.

There is the taste of fresh corn in the fields and the sweet smell of fresh tobacco. For many corn is something you see at the store and tobacco is something in packs. But, I remember the tobacco and corn fields before the crops were cut for marketing. They held great memories because they were great playgrounds for playing games like tag and hide and seek.

There's the adventure of going to the store with the older kids. In a farm community you had to walk what seemed like miles to the store. You stopped everywhere along the way talking to everyone, eating berries, and picking apples off trees. Afterwards there was the excitement of my grandfather coming home from work he always had something in his lunch for us younger kids.

At home with my parents was just as much fun. In the evenings I would collect worms so my father and I could go fishing and anything caught was cooked. One day we had fried fish and the next day there was catfish stew or maybe eel. There was parades in downtown Washington or the trips to Museums. I was really fascinated by the F.B.I. building and the national aquarium. Going to all these places gave me a chance to see things that I would never see in ordinary life. The excitement of going to the beach. Even though I couldn't swim I loved playing in the water. And as a child the pleasure of riding on the train.

After joining the Navy the memory of my first ship. It was an Aircraft carrier. I was amazed at how something so large could float. The experience of being able to swim in the shark filled waters off Vietnam and later shrimping in Alaska. The pleasure of meeting my family at the pier in Athens Greece. The adventure of taking my family to England for vacation. We flew to England on an Air Force cargo plane. What pleasant memories.

There is the excitement of running my first foot Race. I was 39 years old when I started running. I started running a couple of blocks gradually working my body up to 6 miles. My first 6 mile race was in Herring, North Carolina. This was a gruesome cross country race down dirt roads, through corn fields, across sandy beaches and the end was down a paved street. This race I will never forget because I came in last. Finishing this race made me more determine to run better. Through regular training I eventually worked my way up to running in the 13 mile race at William and Mary College. Although I never won a race I learn that many times it's not always coming in first that count, but, more important completing what you start.

WELCOME TO WARREN ELECTRIC

Welcome to WARREN ELECTRIC. Yes this is my world, the world of imagination and ingenuity. Cancer is always attempting to raise its ugly head, my back ache, I have bone pain, and I find myself stressed out often by everyone including relatives, but I'm getting better, SMILE. Here I can try almost anything. Having retired from the navy as a Chief electrician in 1982 having served 21 years and working for various electrical companies and businesses, I started Warren Electric. I started WARREN ELECTRIC in January 1990 with my last paycheck from a company called Positively Electric and my tools. As a business WARREN ELECTRIC working with other associate contractors has worked on many structures commercial and residential. This includes new construction or remodeling. We have also performed emergency repairs and troubleshooting.

WARREN ELECTRIC has worked on a variety of projects. Our largest was a nine-unit apartment complex constructed by O. C. E. developers of Oakland, California. Our largest commercial project was the installation of wiring for computer and printer stations for Graphic land Inc. a large sign making company in Oakland California. This also included the wiring of a printer clean room for their large 3M commercial printer. Another project was THE ENDLESS POOL, this was a special exercise pool where the water moves continually. The project was constructed by Willson/Bailey. My most difficult project was the Endless Pool and that was because it was done shortly after my Bone marrow Transplant. My wife assisted me with the wire installation and a plumber installed the pumps and motors. With our access to parts, material, and technical advise provided by our many suppliers Warren Electric has never failed to complete a project. We provide Quality Material, installation, and friendly service. I've found that my only limitations are funding and lack of paperwork support. Both area's I'm lacking in. It's great having idea but sometimes I say why have ideas when many times there is no one to motivate or encourage you. I've talk to people about my ideas and they make suggestion and say you will get results, and this is a true statement if you're any color but black. I've done everything and tried everything and all I find is that people mainly want to get into your pocket. To get funding you need someone to assist you, to try and organize your paperwork and to do that you need funding, it's a vicious circle people in the business work. Why can't many Blacks get those profitable bids it's mostly color, but many say it's bonding, insurance, and funding. Very few will say experience. It's back to that old thing of funding and paperwork, basic support your business need for success. If your business is to succeed you need those basic requirements, and when you are ill you really need that support.

What do you do when confronted with these problems or situations? You deal with each as they approach you, understanding that some problems you can solve and with others you need some type of support.

I've notice that many view my businesses as folly, but, I don't and when looking down the road five or 10 years I want my business to be a success, but that can't be done without support. Since having cancer things have slowed down, but the ideas keep rolling. I've advertised, and networked with other contractors.

One of my favorite ideas is electrical sales and research or better yet a manufacture technical library. The biggest hang-up is financial funding. A technical library is an outstanding idea because things change every day, equipment becomes obsolete and when this happens people need resources to turn to when they need help. This could mean anything from blueprints for buildings to technical information for high tech equipment. To make information available you must charge customers a fee because in some instances you will have to perform some research, and this means overhead. There is a lot of traveling and networking and this is another necessary expense. How much is needed I would say about a $250,000.00 minimum

Is a technical library possible? Yes. The military has been operating a technical library for at least 50 years to keep all that equipment and weapons operating. Manufacturers have gone out of business but the technical specifications are still needed. The military continue to change, and an up to date and an efficient library is needed. Who is up to the task? *The ideas just keep on coming, what's next?*

BUSINESS

How do you see yourself as a business? What types of images are you giving or attempting to give? Do you take your business seriously?

Myself, I try to view my business seriously, because it represents me. To insure my business run's properly I invest in equipment, parts, computers, software and uniforms, everything to make my business successful. But I find that many times, it's not I and what I think of my business, but peoples own view of me and my business. Many of my customers see my business as something positive, and they like the quality of my work and the price. But there are those who see me as cheap Black labor and many blacks see themselves in the same way. Many believe that Black business should perform work at cost.

Many of our businesses fail because we aren't encouraged to be profitable quite often we're forced out of business. As a contractor I've found that many times people will hire you to perform work and when the job is completed refuse to pay you for services rendered. To get your money you must go through all legal means possible even then you may lose. All this exhaust your working capitol forcing you out of business. Many people want a deal, and when they see you doing well they go to another business, because in their minds they say you're charging too much. But they still want quality.

Many times people want me to do business at cost and to this I must say no because if I continually did so I would go out of business. They want me to buy from business such as Home Depot and charge Home

Depot prices and perform the work at laborer rates. They are never concerned about my research time for an item or the time and gas consumed to obtain the item they believe you must absorb all expenses. Have you sat down and thought about simple expense such as gas? In many instances I've spend as much as $20 in two days. In a year that adds up to quite an expense, so as a business I don't perform work for free. Customers must also realize that when you pay for quality work you're paying for training, education, customer service, and that important guarantee. But if they don't want quality then hire someone off the street.

When operating a business there are some things that we business people must view seriously and be included in the price of product and/or services? They are Overhead and Profit.

a OVERHEAD-Rent, Telephone, Computers and Computer support, Office supplies, Gas, Heat, Electric, Office Personnel, Insurance, Bonding. Example-That credit card service can cost you $30-$40 a month.

a PROFIT-Profit is what's left after paying all expenses. Profit is the return on your business investment and your business is an investment. Do you have ideas and dreams? Profit is the key to expanding, further educating you and your staff, buying new equipment. Without profit your business can't grow.

Some people think that as soon as they get some money from a task or sale that the money is all theirs (My Money) forgetting about overhead expenses. When they run into a financial problem, the first thing they say is what's wrong because I made plenty of money. The problem is you forgot about everything else.

As Blacks dealing with people in today's world many of us ask people to give us something, this is not by accident this is by design, dating from slavery. We have always been placed in a position where we must ask people to give us something, even something that has been earned through agreement or law. We are taught to envy people who achieve great success and wealth, but we allow ourselves to feel guilty when we attempt to achieve those same goals. It seems that quite often people teach us we should stay where we are and let someone else run the show. To this I say I DON'T THINK SO. So as a Black businessman I strive for success.

COMPETITION

Competition is fun and healthy but sometimes it can be a nuisance. What does being sick have to do with competition? My illness is the other team trying to get control of my body. And if they win you know the results. And like anything competitive sometimes the odds are stacked against me. What are some of these things?

$ I could have a bum doctor

$ The food I eat or drink

$ Your social and economical environment

$ Sometimes your mental state may change

$ Sometimes the extent of your illness will have an effect on you.

As in anything competitive you prepare to win by removing or changing those things that can hurt you. I remember early in my treatment I requested that my doctor be changed and he was and that was one my best moves because my new doctor gave me better treatment and medication. And with this change shortly thereafter I received my bone marrow transplant, and my quality of life improved.

Being in business I find that I still deal with competition and I like it. When dealing with competition you find you must be innovative and willing to deal with new ideas. You learn to work with ideas from all directions and experience with certain problems encourage you to seek and utilize new ideas. With a little foresight you work with the ones that best suit your needs. Sometimes after analysis the ideas that you though were foolish are your best answer. As business people my wife and I found that to get new customers and keep old ones we must have good prices and services. Sometimes that's not enough. In today's business world you learn to work with the latest technology and equipment, with the latest equipment it gives you accessibility to a wider market. You find that you also must network. You meet people talk and communicate. No one knows you if you don't wave that flag saying I'm over here.

Many see our businesses and want us to see our businesses as folly. Many of us don't and when looking down the road 5 or 10 years from now we want our businesses to be large but that can't be done without support. I've learned that with every request there is a reason to say NO. In fighting cancer I find that I must confront negative social and economical attitudes, changing equipment and technology, cost and funding. Are you one of those people afraid of competition or challenges, always waiting for someone to always give you something, where you don't have to exert any effort always waiting always begging. To beat cancer you must always show you're the better and a more dynamic force with a positive outlook you will win and beat the competition.

SATISFIED CUSTOMERS

Even when you're sick it's great to know you have satisfied customers. I'm still out there hustling trying to develop the dream of having my own successful business. Even though there are many things that I'm unable to do I still network and meet people. One of the many things to keeping well is being busy with things you like. Do things you like, not what others think you should do. Recently a customer of mines had a

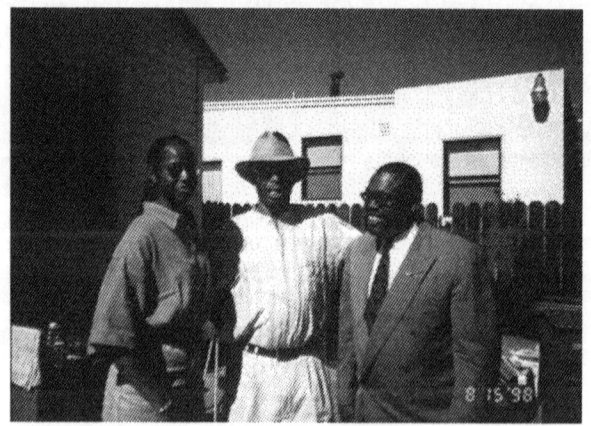

housewarming and she invited my wife and I. While there I developed some new contacts and met some of my old customers. By giving your customers good service and networking it helps to guarantee you future business. Even during my cancer treatments customers were trying to keep me busy. And if they weren't finding work we would discuss future projects.

Remember that in times of great hardship, pain and suffering you don't start withdrawing into yourself, detaching yourself from everyone. You face your problems head on, first recognizing your problem then start working on a solution, but never letting your problems get between you and your friends or your business customers. Develop a relationship with your customers and the people around you.

So if you are sick don't quit, but develop those new ideas. By keeping active you keep you and your customer happy. Instead of worrying about the competition and your health just be concern let everyone else worry while you play to win.

SELF

Are you one of those that are afraid to worry about yourself. Afraid to put yourself and your ideas first. Many times I've had ideas and I tried to sell those ideas and explain how everyone working with me would profits and quite often many would turn things around and would say all I worry about is myself and how selfish I am. And you know that the truth is that I am concern about myself, but selfish I am not, because if you don't push your ideas and dreams who will.

Many times I've attempted to work with others helping them to grow utilizing the training and experience I had been given, knowing my exposure in their business or effort would also help me down the road ,and I find myself and my business being made to look like the villains, when I've made my role as one of assistant. I believe many are afraid to make that commitment to help you, and that attitude to shown when you sit down and talk with them, because they attempt to put you on the defensive. Sure I'm thinking of myself when I discuss subjects and project. I don't like my present position especially that of being sick, but I also believe that I don't have to accept the negative status heaped upon me because I'm a cancer patient or black. For us blacks our getting support for new ideas is very hard because many are comfortable with blacks only in certain fields or job or management levels. We are being held back mentally and economically through teaching. It's amazing how we can get support for operating of non-profit groups or agencies, it's as if people don't mine seeing blacks as beggars. But when we attempt to leave that position then watch out everyone says we're thinking of nothing but ourselves. It appears we aren't doing anything correct if we aren't doing it for free. Many times people want you to give in to their ideas and beliefs before they give you anything. The thing to remember is to believe in yourself and your ideas and understand that putting yourself first many times is not a selfish act and believing in yourself not always in others sometimes is necessary for positive growth and mental healing.

FAITH

How strong is your faith? Going through this fight with cancer and especially chemotherapy, surgery and the Bone Marrow Transplant is a fight you can't forget. It tests your belief in yourself and your faith in God. It's nice to believe in the doctors, herbs and foods, but that's not enough! You need faith to hold everything together; to give you a sense of direction or purpose.

Have you gone through life feeling blessed? Many times I've felt that someone is watching over me. Sometimes I feel as if I'm an angel that has lost a wing. Sure it may sound foolish but I feel some times that I had wings and for some reason I lost mines, but God still looks out for me. Recently I had a dream that if I laid in bed and grabbed the mattress tight that I would develop enough power to make myself rise into the air. I've have dreams many times where I would be able to fly. Sure it's only a dream and I don't think I'm going to die anytime soon. But I do believe God is letting me know he's watching over me and especially though this fight with cancer he's letting me know he's a powerful God. To me it's a blessing to know that I have someone to lean on. when everything seems to go wrong, your problems become so heavy you don't know what to do, you find that nothing seems to go right, wow, it's nice to know you have someone who care.

I look back at my life over the last ten years and the turbulence that was there and how I got through everything without turning to alcohol or drugs. I would have to say it was the power of God that steered me through everything. When I was going through a financial crisis he watched over me. When I had family problems he was there, and in my greatest challenge fighting cancer I feel I have a friend in Jesus and he was my greatest comforter.

Do I believe what I say? The answer is yes. My wife drove me to the hospital emergency room because I was bleeding to death internally and on arrival the doctors and medic's had tubes put down my throat to flush the blood from my stomach and when they went to take blood from me for test they couldn't find my veins and when they eventually drew blood it was clotting so fast that they could hold the tubes upside down and the blood wouldn't flow. To me that was God letting me know he was at work healing my body. I was later told that I had Gastro Intestinal Reflex Disorder (rupture of blood vessels in the stomach) which can sometimes prove fatal. After 3 days of treatment I was discharged from the hospital and a week later I felt as if nothing had happened. One of my neighbors told me he don't know how I recover so fast and I have to smile because I know.

Since having cancer many of my new friends that I met in the cancer program have died. Even some of those that went through the Bone Marrow Program with me have died or their bodies have reject the treatment and now they must take pain pills. Some lost limbs or parts of their body. Your mind go through a lot when see grown healthy people start losing weigh and shrink down to nothing eventually dying or their pain become so great that they have to take some type of narcotic. God has blessed me to not go through all the misery and discomfort, I haven't had any broken bones because of cancer and all the test since having the transplant show no new cancer, and to me that's a blessing. The only medication I take is for controlling my stomach acid and my other pills are vitamins and minerals.

A lot of people say I have changed since going through the transplant at first I said no, but as I progress through recover I find that there are changes going on all the time. Something's I see differently, many things that annoyed me before bother me even more now especially things I see as foolish and destructive. God has got a plan and I'll find out what it is because I may have lost a wing somewhere but Gods eye is on the sparrow so I know he's watching me. If you're having problems put your faith in God because he's the healer, the mediator, the greatest problem solver.

My First Christmas

Yes it's my first Christmas since my transplant and to me it's a great milestone. My wife and grandsons bought a Christmas tree and put on the decorations. On Christmas day we went to my Father-in Laws for dinner. Him and my Mother-in-Law cooked a nice spread. We had turkey ,ham, greens, macaroni and cheese, 2 pies, 2 cakes ,and there was plenty of salads. I tried to eat everything. Afterwards we exchanged gifts I was taking pictures of everyone.

My nephew and his wife was there with their kids including their new baby. The younger nephews and my grandchildren were all over the place with their new toys and when not playing with their toys they were playing with their video games. Everyone had a nice time. I enjoyed everything the most because I think about where I was at the beginning of the year. I thank God for the blessing because I've come along ways. I firmly believe God is smiling on me.

WHEW! TIME REALLY FLIES

It's amazing how quickly time pass. It has been a year and a half since my transplant and things are looking good. You never really consider time and

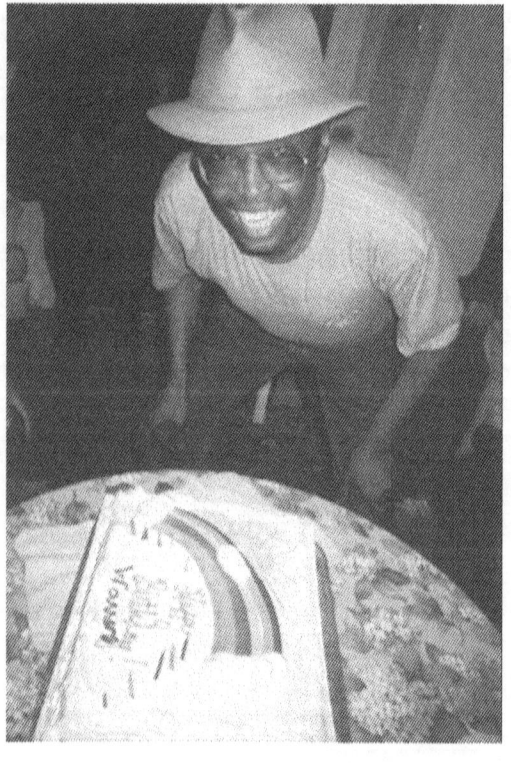

before you know it something reminds you of time. I just celebrated my 55th birthday and it is nice to have reached this point. This is my second birthday since the transplant and the feeling is great. My cousin Joan called from Clinton Maryland and we talked a long time. To help me celebrate, my son and his family came down from Washington State to be with me and they stay four days. It seemed like only yesterday when he was helping me in the hospital and now here he is helping me celebrate another year.

On my birthday my wife, daughter, and granddaughters prepared an authentic Greek dinner and it was fantastic. They prepared stuffed grape leaves, lemon baked chicken, stuffed tomatoes, stuffed squash, spanakopita (spinach and feta cheese pie), Italian sausage soup and baked potatoes. And for Dessert Frances prepared Baklava. The only thing missing was Greek ouzo(liquer) and retsina(wine).

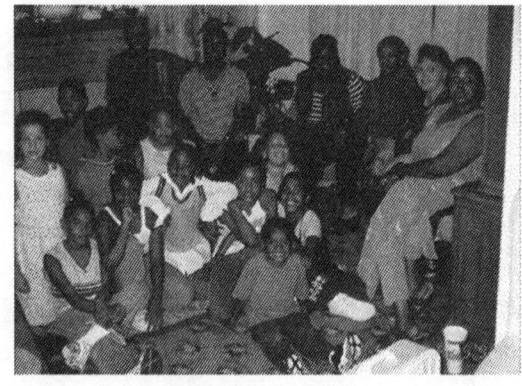

The next day the family members here in Oakland and Richmond had a birthday party for me and it was fantastic. There was kids everywhere and the supply of food was never ending. The house was filled with people. And there was the birthday cake with me blowing out the candles. The complete occasion was something to remember, and I took pictures of everything. So now all I can say is **HAPPY BIRTHDAY.**

CHALLENGE

Challenge—Anything that calls for a special effort.

Do you feel that in fighting cancer that these changes in your life are driving you nuts or more simply put "Driving You up a Wire"?

How many times have you been confronted by something that required you to put that extra effort forward to win or complete a task? These are challenges that when successfully confronted set you apart from everyone. People take notice of what you're doing; they try to get you on their team, sometimes not always for what you would consider good reasons, but they are looking at the positive result of having you with them. Never stop facing those challenges because they are character builders.

Challenges we all must face:

- Family
- Friends
- Jobs
- Business
- Education
- Medical, Etc.

I find challenges are always there, I resolve one and then something else pops up. Sometimes I ask myself what's going on, is something or some-one out there in the world trying to see how much pressure I can take? How many times have we started something but never completed the task, giving up because we believe things are too rough? Forgetting that the preparation is sometimes harder then the task.

Instead of striving for success, are you constantly giving yourself reasons to fail. Set back and really look at yourself. Look at where you're at now and where you want to be 10 or 20 years into the future. Look at why you haven't achieved your goals and if you look at yourself honestly you'll make some fascinating discoveries. All of us have the potential to succeed but many times its something we alone must strive to achieve. Remember the Challenge is not always in winning, but in finishing. Don't be afraid to face those fears, and go after those dreams.

In my efforts success and win in this fight with cancer things are looking better, test results are coming back good. Test results are looking better everyday but what about those problems related to cancer and its treatment that tend to hang on. These are some of the problems:

Lost of stamina-if I work 3 or 4 hours sometimes less, I find I have to stop

! Uncontrollable moments of fatigue.

! Even though I walk at every opportunity, I find walking uphill a scary exercise of mind and body. My heart starts beating like crazy, and my breathing gets heavy or should I say desperate. When I get home I must lay down and rest or take quick nap

! Severe cramping-cramping in my legs, hips and hands

! failing eye site-my vision is becoming worse

! I can't lift heavy objects

! I can't run because the impact bothers the lower section of my legs

! My skin is sensitive to sun light and I must use sun bloke

! Because of all the chemo treatments I now have a sensitive stomach

! Experiencing sharp pains in my right forearm and elbow

! Because of thinning and brittle bones (Osteoporosis) from taking Chemotherapy I must now take a 4 hour treatment of Aredia, which strengthen the bones and prevent the lose of calcium

! I've been admitted to emergency for internal bleeding (gastro intestinal disorder

! I've been admitted for swelling and blood in my knee's

! When I speak about this to people everyone says it age, but I disagree because there are two differences between me and the normal person, Number 1—I have Cancer, and Number 2—I have survived a Bone Marrow Transplant.

! Recently I became ill. I contracted some type of virus that left me with a fever, loss of energy, plus I loss 16 lbs. I was so weak I fainted while getting a chest X-ray. The doctor's told my wife I had some type bronchial infection, Yea, I wonder

As I go through recovery and talk with my fellow Transplant survivors I've learn that I can't take anything for granted not even the smallest thing. I'm now being treated by the Dental team at Travis Air Force Base, David Grant medical center for problems associated with cancer and its treatment. The complete treatment has been exhausting. I'm now scheduled for a Neuro-Psychological Profile test for the Side-effects of Busulfan. When I sleep I find that it takes an effort to awaken. Many times I'm frighten when I'm asleep because I find I have no control over my muscles and I must work to make my muscles respond. Sometimes I find myself feeling as if I'm choking and I must force myself to change position or awaken to clear my breathing. Sometimes I find myself dreaming in a dream. Going through recover is a lot of work. To me Cancer is my greatest challenge and to win I must prepare myself spiritually, physically and mentally. The Bone Marrow Transplant although a challenge is a minor step in winning. I refuse to allow cancer or people to pull me down. I'll meet these problems with a foundation based on faith.

I TIMOTHY 4th Chapter 17th verse-Not withstanding the Lord stood with me, and strengthened me.

I've learned from this horrifying experience of having cancer (a disease that plays on your emotions and that of your family). With Multiple Myeloma your bones can become brittle and break easily. You can develop tumors and lesions. So far I've experienced none of these problem. This does not include the times I was placed in the hospital for having temperatures as high 104 degrees. Or the emergency surgery I had because I developed a blood clot in my neck. Or the blood infection I had; the doctors could not find the source so they had to call in a specialist from the Center for Disease Control, to find out what was wrong and to administer the proper antibiotic to fight the infection. You can't tell me there isn't a God watching over me. Many of my fellow patients were held together with pins or found themselves two or three inches shorter. Some developed tumors, which meant they had to go through Radiation therapy. Even after all the Chemotherapy, Radiation, Surgery and the Transplant a lot of my friends died. This is an unnerving experience.

Many times when my wife wasn't around I would sit on the sofa at home and cry, never asking why me. I would kneel down and pray and ask the Lord to work with me. I've learned not to dwell on how I got the disease or the people that were in charge when I contracted the disease, that just leads to inner bitterness and hatred, which creates negative emotions and in fighting cancer that can be destructive. During the chemotherapy treatments and the Bone Marrow Program my wife was with me, she accompanied me to the hospitals, and in many instances she slept in the room with me. The times when I passed out she was there, never complaining but comforting me and when things got really tough we would hold hands and pray. You learn to never give up believing in yourself and having faith in God because you are going to have serious problems, financial, medical and spiritual all through this program, but with Gods help you can make it through.

A HERO IS GONE

A piece of Anacostia, Washington D.C. has died.

His name was Warren Gamaliel Harding Fisher, a.k.a Fabulous Fisher, he was my father. He died 7 October 1999.

In a time when many people seem to be bringing down the image of the Black male here was a true hero. Even after losing his sight he still attempted to be involved in everything. As a parent he taught me writing skills, my sister he taught organizational skills and my brother well he learned music. Born March 14, 1921 to Carrie Fisher of Washington D.C. and Alexander Piner of Chestertown Maryland in Kent county. Born and raise in the southwest community of Washington D.C., but after completing his military service in May 1946 he moved his family to the Black community of Anacostia.

His ambition was to always write. This interest started while attending the Paul Lawrence Dunbar High School in Washington D.C.. He graduated as an honor student in 1939. His writing and journalist skills were later enhanced during his time in the service. After separating from the Army he held numerous jobs finally being employed by the Defense Department as a clerk. He worked in numerous locations including the pentagon. Because he was always interested in the Black community he wrote many articles and took many picture of the Black community. In the forties and fifties he followed the Black athletics clubs like the football team Anacostia Troopers and the baseball team Anacostia A.C.. And he kept you up to date with the city night life. Although never hired by the white media he wrote for many of the Black publications and this included the Washington Spotlight, Washington Informer, and the Washington Afro American. In the informer his column was Across The River with Fab Fisher, Anacostia Southeast. Here he kept you up to date with all the current events, and that was political and social. He also became a noted photographer tracking the communities history with all its ups and downs through his pictures. He had photographs of the parades, athletic teams, the kids in the junior police boys club and the Black theater.

Here was a man who was everywhere. While working for the government and writing he still had time to operate two businesses. Him and his long time friend Reverend E.W. Stevenson co-founded A.P. Shaw United

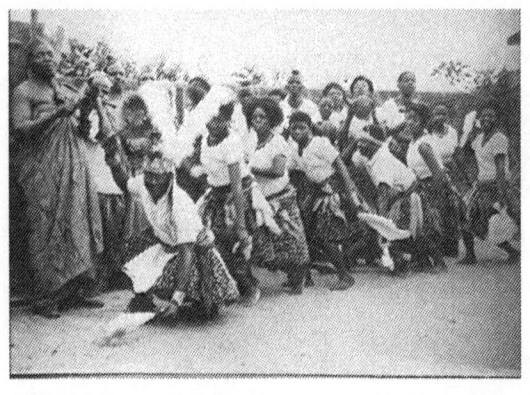

Methodist Church which is still a permanent land mark in Anacostia. Here he played the piano, directed the choir, helped organize church plays and other social events.

Another of his interest was Africa. Fluent in many languages, by 1962 he was the host to as many as 250 African students. In December 1962 the Washington Daily News wrote an article stating that he was a ONE MAN STATE DEPARTMENT.. The Anacostia Business and Professional association said he knew more French speaking Africans than anyone in Washington D.C.. He even adopted some of the African students from the African Republic of Mali, and there were children named in his honor.

Many of his photographs documenting the history of Anacostia and his involvement with African students were placed on display at the Smithsonian Carver Theater museum located in Anacostia. Some of his photographs were also placed on display at the American Embassy in

Leopoldville in the Congo. Much of his involvement in community, politic's, and social event's was done without outside financial support, many times his only support was his ingenuity.

Always trying to educate he took my sister, brother and myself on numerous trips to places like New York, Philadelphia, New Jersey, and Baltimore visiting museums and historic landmarks. Always striving and on the move he kept track of everyone, family and friends. You could always expect to receive a card from him on all holidays and birthdays.

Oh the memories. Many of us forget what our parents have done, only thinking of those monetary rewards. For me, my father left memories in pictures and stories and the ability to observe and enjoy my surroundings. If we all look beyond our selfish desires what pleasant memories we will find and the excitement of those memories.

Now gone he will be missed, a hero to many of us.

Fabs Thanks

Fabulous Fisher, April 2, 1981

Fab thanks God for folks like you!
I was sixty years old on my last birthday
Unfortunately, I celebrated my
birthdays in Washington Hospital
Center. I walked out alone but not really
alone because my hand rested in
God's hand. He blessed me to
come out strong and fabulously
to do my thing which is Sharing
God's blessings with you and
all others. Fab can help...

We people-Black or White, Negro or Colored, Jew or Gentile, Young or old, straight or Gay, Saint or Sinner or even Alcoholic or Teetotaler...

We all need God's help in this
ridiculously psychedelic era in
which we are fortunate to live in.

If you are a senior or middle
age person, you have *experience.*
**SHARE THAT EXPERIENCE WITH THE
YOUNGSTERS AND YOUNG ADULTS WHO THINK THE
PRINCIPLES OF LIFE ARE EASY TO COME BY...**

Don't think that Fab Fisher
is really crazy and spend thrifty
to send out all these cards
to you and many folks like you.
I, Warren Fisher, known to
all under the pen name of
Fabulous Fisher alias Fab
loves the idea of remembering
as many people as I can while
they are around and it always
gives me a great feeling of
seeing flowers given to the
living. God and his loving
Son Jesus Christ have blessed
all of us be here and I
am simply saying in the teachings
of Christ **Share your blessings
with others because it keeps
us all enthused to**
KEEP ON KEEPING ON
                FAB

It's Tough Trying to Survive in Today's World

It's tough trying to survive in today's world. Everyone is being tossed about mentally and physically. In the need to survive and get ahead there is still that self destructive nature of man. It seems that in order to succeed you must destroy everything in sight. There is no concern about anything or anyone as long as you achieve your desires. There is that consume everything attitude and if something can't be eaten than you destroy it. This includes not only material, but there is also that destruction of people. The sad thing about all this is that many will destroyed themselves just to please or get attention from others.

As I move about I find a sometimes changing time in peoples attitude, life style and imaginary skills. How did those Blacks in the past get ahead. Their education level were equal or in many cases were better than whites, but their access to the system was limited and in many instances nil. Intimidation from outside the community was expected. The thing they learned and taught was survival and adaptability technics. They took what was placed in front of them and they made everything work. With this they built some impressive communities.

Now the Black community is changing and many are deteriorating. Now we are being taught to question ourselves and our very legal existence. We have been taught to debate. There is nothing wrong with debating. But do we have to stop an debate an issue before making a decision? We must learn to debate and make serious decision while on the move. When the machine stops to have a debate so does everything else. It's funny we're stopping to debate issues while the system is still moving and instead of building more institutions of higher learning are building more prisons to house more Black prisoners. When we stop to debate we now become distracted from the main issues and many will use this opportunity to put us in positions we normally wouldn't allow. In these debates many times we allow ourselves to be treated as adolescents, as a social group we still consider ourselves adolescence and now we must let people know we are tired of being treated that way. We must learn to be the manipulator and not the manipulated. Like adolescents we think of images and pleasant times in the old neighborhood what people now call the hood. These were images basically from childhood in a community or housing project where there was no ownership, where your life in essence was controlled or governed by others. Many forget the effort and struggle their parents endured in creating these pleasant communities with the resources available. Everyone claims they love the hood but when they get angry with someone the first thing they destroy is the hood.

Now everyone is talking about what everyone should be doing for them. Many forget or have that selective memory about what their forefathers endured in order for them to have a better future. Like blood suckers instead of enhancing what was left, they consume. I remember going into a house where the mother is busy working and her unemployed not unemployable sons in their thirties are sitting around with their oversize belly, beers in hand, belching and asking for money for more. Or the house where everyone's main concern is where they can get their next joint. You know where everyone is high and they are all slid down in their seat talking about that good shit. Or the women who have babies and believe the babies are someone else responsibility. And I won't forget the house I went into that was so filthy and smelly that my wife made me take bath once I returned home. There is the house where the father is a drunk and the children and the dog are fighting over the dog food. As I walk through the neighborhood where I was raise in my youth where once stood thriving businesses now stand abandon hulks. Many businesses and housing projects are now boarded up scheduled for demolition. Seeing all this activity you ask yourself, why? These are things you must recognize and remember because here you learn and understand that many don't have the same interest as you.

Look around and you will see a sometimes depressing world. The world doesn't have to be that way, but these are images being imposed on us, all in the name of God or humanity just to justify what is happening. For Blacks the climate is sometimes stressfully. Given full civil rights in the 60's I find full acceptance of us in the American society by many including ourselves is difficult. Many forget that we help build this country, now everyone wants to have that selective memory. We talk about our future and our children's future but what type of world are we creating. Many of us try to be positive and look toward a better future, hey it's hard. Churches talking about the worlds going to end and how we must stop everything and get ready, there is an ever increasing dependence on drugs, airplanes falling from the sky due to poor workmanship or sabotage, kids killing each other (and this includes friends) in school and on the street in the name of some type of hate or for just a plain thrill, and male, female relationship especially in the family is suffering. The list is long, and it appears everyone is trying to give you a reason to fail or why you should accept things as they are.

What can I do about everything, I really don't know? In my world I try to be positive. When confronted with a problem I face it with a I will win type attitude. Because of this attitude I win more than I lose. I put my faith in God and a belief in myself. I want you know that it is tough. I've been in the hospital on numerous occasions, many of my friends and relatives have died, but the will and the need to survive is still there. Many make it appear so easy to give in into that negative side of life. Don't give in because sometimes all you need is the desire to see what is on the other side of hill or around the corner. As a Black many of us have learn that the barriers to growth and improvement are still there. Yea, I know if you work you will get ahead. The question is how far? The truth of the matter is that we still live in a white controlled society. Sure things get done but you must have whites approval. In a truly integrated society you are suppose to have options and Blacks don't have them. What happened to the Black society? For years we had black businesses, Financial institutions, world class education systems. Many of our institutions are gone having been destroyed or limited in their reach through legal manipulation and we've become more dependent on the very society who created the system we live in. Our problem was that we were not given true access to opportunity which means our growth is now stifled. Integration was suppose to solve our problem, but it didn't, instead it created more problems? Now we have become more dependent on the white society. Instead of creating a 2 way economy we still have a one way economy, yes, but we have a few more dollars.

Many of our people have negative attitudes. Why? You are taught so many things and when you get out into the world, you find everything is an illusion to get money out of you pocket, not put anything in your pocket. Look at your businesses no matter how large your business become it is still considered a small business and you believe it. You learn quickly the feeling of rejection and its affects. The question is are you ready to confront these problems? Are you a builder or a consumer? On that highway of life are you one of those who set goals, assigning yourself destination and working to complete your task or are you always hitch-hiking always ready to accept what comes. Ask yourself these questions. Are you a participant or a hitchhiker? Are you a destroyer or disrupter? Are you a consumer or builder? Do you give constructive criticism or are you one of those who argue just for the sake of arguing unconcerned about the answers or results. Many believe everyone owes them something. Many people really believe that it's not what they should do for themselves, but what everyone should do for them. Everyone can deny what I say, but how many times have you heard people say that if no-one will do for them then they are going to continue doing the wrong they have been doing. How self destructing people can be? In a time when Blacks want equal rights and equal justice, we must still teach accountability. Equal rights is not the mimic of others wrong or injustice in the need to advance, when you do this you are not advancing you are moving backward. In our need to get ahead we sometimes embrace the very things we hate. There is the dealing of drugs, hey a little can go along ways, especially 10 years in jail. Many are turning to the gay community thinking that's going to give them more opportunity, if people are uncomfortable associating with you when you're Black, how are things going to change when they find out you're gay and Black. In the need to get money there is the being a front for white business, so they can get minority contracts. You know the drill they use your name and identity to get lucrative multimillion dollar contracts. Hey no sweat, you get all the responsibility and 2% of the contracts and they get the rest. Sometimes we can make some poor choices.

How quickly many forget that Black crime even murder was considered acceptable or even entertaining especially to the white community, giving many Blacks a value of poor self worth. With the acceptability of today's drug culture that vary attitude is still reflected. Children especially we must teach them to understand that just because someone does something wrong and get away with it doesn't justify their doing it. In the end this means that someone has to be accountable. If you do an adult crime expect an adult punishment. Accountability and responsibility is something that should be taught starting at childhood.

Life is complicated with no sure answers but as we move through life we learn and hopefully we grow and with this growth we enhance our future.

Remembrance

For us Blacks in today's fast pace world of high drug use, crime, and greed, we must not allow ourselves to be caught up in the mischief of others. but in our need to advance we must use the teaching of those gone before us to move us through the turbulence of time.

WELCOME TO THE CAFÉ

Warren G.H. Fisher Jr

Hey, Welcome to the Cafe. Deals are being made here every day. What year is this? Well it is 1951. Are you surprised? Look around and it is hard

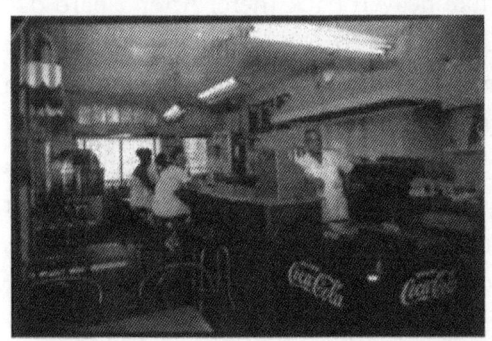

to picture deals being made here. Go ahead walk around check the place out. Check out the ladies at the counter sipping Coca Cola, you know coke is the latest thing. There is suppose to be a hot party going on this weekend, ask the ladies they might know where. While you're doing all that get a ice cold soda water out of the soda machine. Hungry? I recommend the tuna fish or grill cheese sandwiches.

This place is really nice. Here you can sit and listen to the jukebox or on Fridays listen to the fights. Myself, on weekends I like sitting at home with the kids and listening to Lights Out or The Shadow. Those radio people have quite an imagination. Don't like the place, well, we can go to Dr. Quarles pharmacy and soda fountain. Me, I find this place much more comfortable for doing business deals.

So, lets get down to business. I understand you want to start a business. You know it is about time you did something. I see you all the time working a hustle. The only way for Negro's to get ahead is start a business. I wonder what would happen if we were ever equal to whites. Well, it's only a thought. You know the whites would burn down everything rather than see us equal. Those Crackers are really something. I read in the Afro-American just last week the whites lynched a boy for whistling at a white girl. We know he didn't, but those white boy's don't care, because he was just another nigger. Scary world we live in.

Well, back to business. What type of business you want to start? I know you're good with your hands. That's a nice house you and your wife built on 10th street. I really like the back yard, on a cool day you can smell the perfume from those flowers. It's like heaven back there. After a hard day it's a nice place to sit and dream. And you are a great cook. They tell me you learned all that while living in Harlem. Myself, I think you learn everything from watching your grandmother. How is she anyway?

I notice in your new house you now have gas heat. Who helped you build that fancy system? Me, I'm still dealing with the coal furnace. Its not bad, but sometimes you find yourself getting up to a cold house. That's really bad when the temperature outside is really cold and there is 2 feet of snow on the ground.

Hey, here comes Mr. Johnson. He is the person who will work with you. You know Mr. Johnson, small world. Hello Mr. Johnson I believe you know each other. Mr. Johnson, my friend wants to start a business and I believe we can help. Well I'll leave so you can work out the details. I'm going to get myself some ice cream, you know I love that stuff. Call me when you are finished.

Frank, what kind of ice cream you got? I'll try that cherry vanilla and I'll take an orange pop. This ice cream is real good. Did you change company's or what? Let me have a couple of those El Producto cigars. I'll smoke them at the office. Frank, how are the twins doing, I know they are growing fast. One of them have a cold. Take him to see Doc. I understand he'll be working late today. I see that Mr. Johnson is finish conducting business, back to work. I'll talk at you later.

Mr. Johnson, I see you have finished and I believe everyone is satisfied. Tomorrow everyone come to my office and I'll have all the paperwork ready. Mr. Johnson, I know you have to go, time waits for no-one.

Well, mister business man what do you think? The money is guaranteed to be in your hands tomorrow. Surprised? I bet you were thinking you had to see those white bankers in their fancy suits. Hey, that won't happen because they are afraid of us colors as competition. This is how most of our colored businesses develop. If I make money you make money, If you make money I make money. It's that old saying one hand feeds the other.

Whew, I'm tired. I been busy today running 3 businesses, and now that I'm finished here I'm going home and take it easy. I'll stop and get a bag of cooked crabs and a couple of bottles of beer and while relaxing listen to music from Ella and Duke. I wonder if records will ever be replaced. It's a thought. I'll see you tomorrow.

THROUGH THE EYES OF DREAMERS

Have you ever looked at those old pictures of elderly Black people sitting in that rocker on the front porch, or just sitting on the front stoop of their house and wondered what they were thinking. Looking at how empty their eyes can sometimes look, some with smiles many without. For many now there are no porches or stoops instead they are in

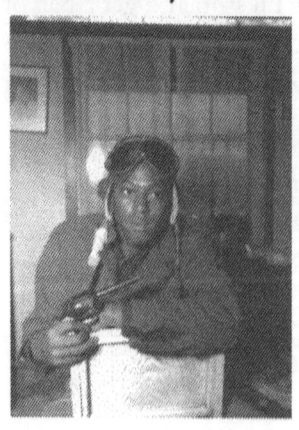 senior homes or in senior centers sitting in a recliner no ambition, no hope, many it appears quietly waiting for death. I sat in my mothers chair and the feel was scary. That chair appeared to be drawing the life force out of me. I felt I was aging quite rapidly. Is this what we must look to when growing old? I believe this is something that doesn't have to happen. Aging is a natural process, but at what point is old? Mentally people can be so cruel to each other. Looking thru those old photographs many made by my father a man who tracked Black history of the family and the community I can see what my father saw thru his eyes.

Though he eventually became blind I still had an opportunity to see the Black world as he saw it. Here was not a world as we view it on Television, but the true Black community in the forties and fifties. This was the world of the dreamers. People who not only saw the future, but

felt we should be part of that future. These weren't people looking for an easy ride, but laborers, housekeepers, garbage and trash collectors, teachers, doctors, lawyers, builders of every type attempting to become part of the American dream. They saw the prosperity of the future, but found themselves being denied true access to that prosperity. Here true accomplishments was way beyond their reach. Accomplishments that many today refuse to recognize or accept.

What has those eye's seen? Yes, there is the cruel side of our nation. There is the years of being denied the rights to intellectual property, where 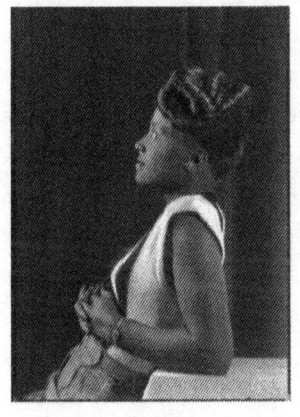 your thinking and imagination is suffocated, over 40 years of no political representation. But, looking thru those eyes you see Blacks dreaming and attempting to create a future. There is the young children and the young adults they taught, the businesses they created. The young men dreaming and working toward success. The women building dignity and style unmatched. There are the athletic teams, and culture classes. These are all part of a village attempting to build a nation.

Now when I see the sad faces of the elderly, I wonder if they are sad because of disappointment. Many of the dreams our elders built whether social, business, or political, instead of investing, expanding and enhancing , we have abandon or sold. Instead of continually striving for success many of us have settle for the crumbs. Many forget that true success can not come without struggle and sacrifice. Our elderly accomplished much, they fought in every war, and helped build this great society and now how tired and worn many are ,because the burden has become so great. **So think of those elderly and ask do you want your future to be their past and their struggle to build a nation lost?**

AM I MY MOTHER'S CHILD

Am I my mothers child? Sometimes I feel like I'm a hundred years old. I've been many places and done many things. For many, they claim they don't remember I guess I'm unusual because I remember almost everything. In the forties I remember my father giving me a green Donald Duck jacket

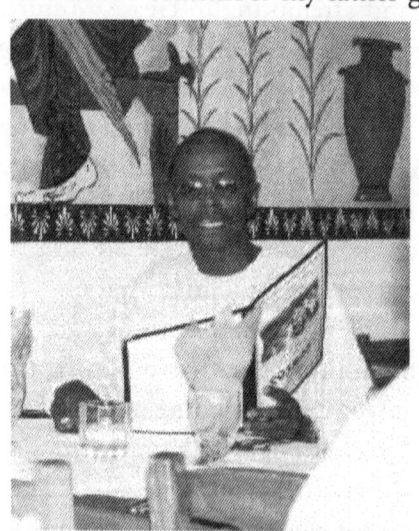 and I loved that jacket. I remember the parades in Washington D.C. along tree lined Pennsylvania and Constitution Avenue, the trees were later cut down because of some type of fungus. The smell of Diesel fumes from those buses as they moved about the city. The sound of electric Street Cars moving about on their tracks and the sound of overhead sparking wires as they moved along the street. This was a time when you didn't have automated street lights. At the corner of 7th and Pennsylvania Ave there was a policeman in a booth high above the street controlling the traffic lights during rush hour. Today you see people pushing grocery carts collecting cans and bottles trying to make money. In the 40's and early 50's many couldn't afford cars and trucks so they used horse and wagon to move about town to collect junk to sell to the local junk yards. Many

homes didn't have central heating, they were heated by kerosene, wood, or coal. I remember the kerosene truck making it's weekly visit to our neighborhood. Television was the big thing. My parents first television was a Jackson with a 17" screen. There was only four television stations and I tried to watch everything. A real luxury was the refrigerator, because many people could only afford a ice box. The popular soft drinks were Coca Cola, Pepsi, Nehi, Royal Crown, and Rock Creek. The popular beers were Budweiser, Miller, Pabst Blue Ribbon, and Balentine

At six I remember my mother putting me on the bus by myself to go to my Aunt Ross house in southwest. She would tell the bus driver where I was going and the drivers on each bus insured I got there. My first trip to the dentist was at Turner Elementary School and getting my immunization shots at D. C. General Hospital and Freeman Hospital, and Steel braces being attached to my legs at Dr Hadleys Children Hospital because I had deformed legs. That John Deere tractor my grandfather bought with its steel wheels and really being excited when he finally bought a tractor with rubber tires. Riding in my grandfathers 1940's ford and my fathers first car a green 1956 Dodge I fondly called Bessie. I remember my cousins living at 220 K Street, Southwest Washington D.C. This was a family of 7 living in a 2 bedroom house. Although they had running water, lights and gas the toilet was outside in the backyard. The family celebrated the Holidays as a family unit. Easter we were at my grandparents, Thanksgiving at my Aunt Tippy's and Christmas at my parents home. That was when everyone caught-up on the latest gossip.

As time moved on, Bus tickets for school were a dime. To go to the movie was thirty five cents and to see a premier movie was a dollar fifty. My father encouraged me to go to the free musical programs at the National Gallery of Art. After the United States entered the space program I remember the government putting a building on Pennsylvania Ave filled with computers which you could view from the street letting us see our space program at work. I remember cars like the Packard, Hudson, Studebaker, and the Rambler. And everyone laughing at small cars like the

Volkswagen. I saw the change from the giant UNIVAC computers to the personal computer.

As I grew older I later joined the Navy, got married and with my family I traveled everywhere. In San Diego my wife and I and our two kids lived in a 1 bedroom apartment paying $55.00 a month rent my pay was $150.00 a month, later we moved to Boston with the cold and snow and where we had another child. We moved from Boston to Quincy Massachusetts where we found ourselves working three jobs each and still having time to raise 3 kids. Next we moved to Virginia and on to Greece. We lived in Greece with its sunny beaches, houses with beautiful marble and wood floors. We were there when the Greek Government changed hands three times. There was the dictatorship, Military Junta, and finally a Democratic government. To us Greece was home because my Wife and kids spoke Greek and with the assistance of my kids adopted Greek grandmother it was easy for everyone to adapt to the Greek way of life. During my time in the Navy I saw many changes. There was the change from Crude oil to Nuclear and Gas Turbine (Jet Engines) to power ships. From guns to cruise missile and smart bombs. Although my main trade was as electrician, my collateral duties were race relations, legal rights counselor and assistant education officer. Many of these positions have been discontinued. I've seen the country go from segregation to integration. And after retiring from the Navy I found myself working for families whose grandparents served with the confederate army during the civil war.

It's exciting to have seen all these changes and at times to have participated. Hopefully in the future I will see even more changes and improvements. Now I'm into my eighth year of fighting Cancer, I've survived chemotherapy, a bone marrow transplant and I continually improve.

Am I my mother's child?

Yes, I am my mother's child and my fathers son and the stories just keep coming.

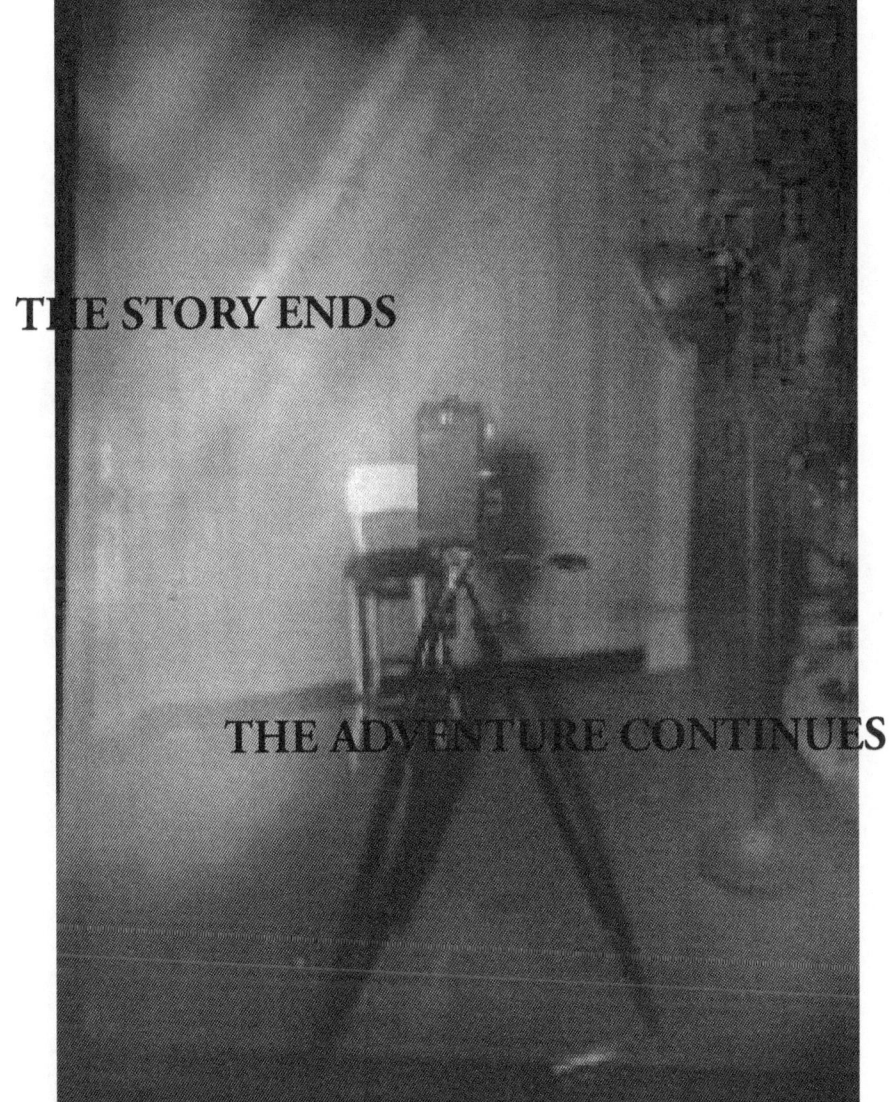

THE STORY ENDS

THE ADVENTURE CONTINUES

www.ingramcontent.com/pod-product-compliance
Lightning Source LLC
Chambersburg PA
CBHW021602280526
45784CB00001BA/473